# Health Services for Tomorrow

# Health Services for Tomorrow

## Trends and Issues

by Eveline M. Burns

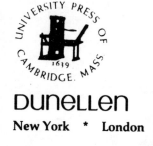

## DUNELLEN

**New York  *  London**

CC

# Contents

## Part 3  1965: A Turning Point

# Preface

Major changes in the financing and delivery of the nation's health services can be expected in the years immediately ahead, and these will inevitably involve a greater role for government. It has now become evident that the strategic policy decisions in these areas can no longer be left to the outcome of the operations of the economic market or the controls exercised by professional and provider organizations. Consumers are dissatisfied with the rising costs of the health services, with the difficulty of finding their way through the uncoordinated maze of providers in their search for continuity of comprehensive, high quality care, with the conditions under which health services are delivered (which seem often to be devised for the convenience and comfort of the providers rather than the recipients), and, in far too many cases, with the nonavailability of needed services due to financial barriers, shortages or maldistribution of providers, or other reasons. Nor is dissatisfaction with existing arrangements confined to consumers. An increasing number of members of the health professions are critical of the status quo because it impedes their ability to render high quality professional service to individuals and prevents the health service industry from contributing the full potential of its scientific knowledge and technological skill to the national well-being.

Numerous proposals for change are now before the nation. Many are highly complex and all present difficult policy choices. I have always believed that in a democracy public policy decisions are likely to be made more rationally and wisely if the electorate is aware of the available alternatives and the issues at stake. It therefore becomes the responsibility of the professional student of social policy to use his expertise to cut through technicalities and details so as to identify major trends and issues and reveal the more important social and economic implications of alternative policies in language that can be understood by the intelligent citizen, whether lay or professional. This I have tried to do.

Part I of this book describes the organization and functioning of the present system (or, as some would say, "nonsystem") and identifies some of the more important developments in the science and technology of medicine and in public attitudes and expectations which have both intensified the problems of the health services and created a demand for change. Central to that demand is the growing conviction that the community, as such, must exercise more influence, or even control, over the manner in which the health services are financed and organized.

In this country, and even more elsewhere, there has been increasing resort to government as the instrument through which that influence can be exerted. Public action can, of course, take many forms and policies can be implemented in a variety of ways. It is thus important that there should be an awareness of the available options and of their potentialities and limitations. Part II therefore surveys the variety of roles which have been assigned to government in this and other countries, and deals in some detail with the three non-means-tested systems for the financing and organization of health services: (1) voluntary publicly subsidized health insurance, (2) compulsory health insurance, and (3) a national health service (the only one of the three that can properly be described as "socialized medicine").

Part III concentrates on the profound changes brought about by the Social Security Amendments of 1965, which enacted Medicare and Medicaid and identifies the major policy issues to which this legislation gave rise.

Part IV looks ahead. It focuses largely on compulsory health insurance proposals, examining them from the point of view of their probable impact, for good or bad, on the many problems that afflict the health services today. These problems are far more extensive and more obdurate than the removal of the financial barrier to receipt of needed services, although this objective, in the United States as elsewhere, has been the primary stimulus to public action. Among them are the need for rationalization of the delivery system, the assurance of an adequate supply and appropriate geographical distribution of institutional, professional and para-professional providers, control of cost escalation, assurance of economical use of the resources devoted to the health services, and the development of an administrative structure that is neither rigidly centralized nor uncontrollably fragmented, that assures accountability and is responsive to consumer interests. The book concludes with a forecast of some probable future developments.

The individual chapters originally appeared as articles or chapters in various publications. Apart from the deletion of introductory or concluding paragraphs which would have meaning only for the audience specifically addressed, the chapters (except for Chapter 10, which has been considerably expanded) are reproduced as originally written. Although they cover a span of years, I have not updated the statistical data given in the earlier chapters, for they provide the context in which they were written, and since in all cases I indicate the date to which the figures apply, there should not be any occasion for confusion. Inevitably, since the papers were addressed to different audiences at different times there is some repetition of themes, and to a lesser degree, of factual material. However, some measure of repetition is inevitable when dealing with so complicated a system as the health services. Many features of the system have a variety of relationships and consequences, and when focusing on any one problem or aspect the reader needs to be reminded of other relevant ramifications. The very fact that people are still struggling with many of the same problems that we have grappled with over a period of years while conveying an implied reproach for our lack of progress also suggests that the problems are complex and difficult and are not to be resolved by any simple or single reform.

I have been emboldened to believe that this kind of analysis of social policy serves a useful purpose by the response to many of my papers. The volume of requests for reprints from health professionals, from teachers, notably in medical and social work schools, and from members of action-oriented civic organizations has for some time been more than I could cope with. Especially encouraging has been the interest shown by many members of the medical profession and by health services experts. I have profited greatly from their writings, from discussions and from joint service on committees, though needless to say, I alone am responsible for errors and omissions. It would be impossible to list all of those who have helped me but it would be ungrateful not to express my indebtedness to some from whom I have received particular encouragement or instruction. Among them are:

Professor Harry Becker, Division of Community Medicine, Albert Einstein College of Medicine, Yeshiva University; Dr. Lester Breslow, M.D., Chairman, Department of Preventive and Social Medicine, University of California, Los Angeles; Dr. Ruth Freeman, R.N., School of Hygiene and Public Health, Johns Hopkins University; Beverlee Myers, Assistant Administrator, Health Services and Mental Health Administration, Department of Health, Education, and Welfare; Professor Nora Piore, School of Public Health and Administrative

Medicine, Columbia University; Professor George Silver, M.D., Yale University; Professor Anne R. Somers, Department of Community Medicine, Rutgers Medical School, Rutgers University; Professor Herman M. Somers, Princeton University; Professor Kerr White, M.D., School of Hygiene and Public Health, Johns Hopkins University; Alonzo S. Yerby, M.D., Harvard School of Public Health; and two who tragically are no longer with us, the late Dr. George James, M.D., former Dean of Mount Sinai School of Medicine, and the late Professor E. Richard Weinerman, M.D., Yale University. And as an economist, I am particularly grateful for the privilege of membership in the Committee on Social Policy for Health Care of the Committee on Special Studies of the New York Academy of Medicine whose deliberations enriched my understanding of the problems of the health services and the points of view of the medical profession and stimulated me into applying the approach I had developed in analyzing income maintenance policies to the field of the health services.

My indebtedness to the various publishers who have given permission for the reproduction of articles is indicated by notes at the beginning of each chapter. Finally, I would like to express my appreciation of the interest and help I have received from Mrs. Paule Jones, Executive Editor, The Dunellen Publishing Company, Inc.

Eveline M. Burns

New York City, December 1972

# PART 1

# THE NEED FOR CHANGE

# 1 Three Revolutions

The inadequacies of the present system for the financing and delivery of personal health services are widely recognized, and although there are strong differences of opinion as to the nature of the remedies, there is a growing consensus that change is long overdue. In fact change is likely to be hastened, and in some respects facilitated, by developments in three areas, whose impact on social policy for health services in the nation as a whole is likely to be so profound as to deserve the epithet "revolutionary." These are the revolutions that have occurred in the realms of social attitudes and values, scientific and technical advances in medicine, and arrangements for the financing of medical care.

## The Revolution in Social Attitudes and Values

It is evident that in recent years the public has come to attach an increased value to health as such. By 1966, the Congress, in passing PL 89-749 (the Comprehensive Health Planning and Public Health Services Amendment Act) could declare: "the fulfillment of our national purpose depends on promoting and assuring the highest level of health attainable for every person, in an environment which contributes positively to healthful individual and family living . . ." This is no mere rhetorical declaration. For it is obvious that the public's expectations in the field of health and its demands on medicine have become increasingly articulate, specific, and insistent.

Originally published under the title "The Challenge and the Potential of the Future," as an appendix to the report entitled *Comprehensive Community Health Services for New York City, Report of the Commission on the Delivery of Personal Health Services.* New York, the Commission, n.d. (written in 1967).

1

There is now wide support for the belief that everyone should have access to the benefits of modern medicine, and Title XIX of the Social Security Act now gives effect to the view that medical care shall not be denied any person merely because he cannot afford to pay for it.

The public demand is also increasingly for continuous and comprehensive care in contrast to the present fragmentation. It follows that future arrangements must assure the availability of primary physician services to all residents and that the primary physician in turn (whether working in solo practice or as a member of a private group or neighborhood health center) must be related to the full spectrum of health resources and in particular to a teaching hospital or medical school, so that his patients may have available to them the full reach of medical knowledge and resources.

The public attitude toward the receipt of health care appears, however, to go further than this, and to concern itself with the circumstances under which this care is available. The demand now is for access to health services to be prompt, convenient, comfortable, and free of offensive or discriminatory conditions.

Satisfaction of these demands will require many changes. It will involve the abandonment of the dual system of personal health services whereby there was one system of care for the comfortable or rich and one, less desirable, for the poor. This change will be hastened by the new financing under Titles XVIII and XIX of the Social Security Act which, by making public funds available to pay the reasonable costs of care of the eligible population (both Medicare and Medicaid) has at a stroke abolished whatever justification there might previously have been for treating the "charity patient" as a second-class patient who was expected to be grateful for whatever treatment he received because much of it was rendered at zero or submarket rates of remuneration by institutional or professional providers. Today there are fewer and fewer "charity patients."

But fragmented, inconvenient, and inconsiderate treatment has not in the past been confined to the poorer patients, and satisfaction of the demand for access for all to needed health services that is prompt, convenient, comfortable, and free of offensive conditions will involve a restructuring of the health services to provide that the point of entry to the total system be geographically convenient and continuously available to all residents. It means transferring the functions of the often inconveniently placed and overloaded hospital outpatient department (and of the emergency room when used as a substitute for more appropriate points of entry to the system) to a series of neighborhood health centers or groups of primary physicians. It calls

2

for an expansion of community-based services and facilities, many of a paramedical nature. It is essentially a demand that the interests and convenience of the patient, rather than of the profession or the institution, shall be decisive.

On the other hand there is a growing public restiveness about the mounting costs of health care and a demand for accountability on the part of the providers of medical goods and services, both in the narrower fiscal sense and in terms of performance, quality, and responsible use of scarce resources. The mystique that hitherto surrounded medicine is decaying, and there will be growing public support for public evaluation of the functioning of the system as a whole, as well as its individual parts, and for the use of controls and sanctions. This attitude will favor the adoption of changes aiming at a more effective structuring of the entire system.

## The Technical and Scientific Revolution

The impact of modern science and technology on the practice of medicine has been spectacular. Refinements of techniques and almost incredible human skill, coupled with the availability of specialized and intricate equipment and the application of new knowledge from the physical as well as the biological and behavioristic sciences, have vastly increased the potential capacity of medicine as a whole.

But remarkable as have been its achievements in regard to specific procedures and the treatment of the individual patient, the application of modern science and technology to the organization and administration of the health services, either as a whole or in various subsystems, has so far lagged behind. From now on, one can expect a more general adoption of modern techniques for storing and retrieving information, for transmitting information, and for imaginative use of the newer methods of communication to facilitate consultation among geographically separated specialists. Automatic devices to facilitate follow-up of patients or identification of needs for further intensive service which so far have been little developed can be expected to become of general use. Automation of diagnostic procedures and laboratory tests is only now beginning to make an impact. Even the computerizing of appropriate aspects of hospital management and administration has not yet been fully exploited.

These developments in information and communication technology, and in automation, and their application to the operation of the health services make available powerful new administrative tools for grappling with some of the problems to which the practice of scientific medicine

3

has given rise. But they are only tools and must be utilized in the framework of specific social policy objectives if the potentialities of modern science and technology are to be realized and if the problems which they have created are to be solved. These problems are numerous and stubborn.

(1) *The rapid advances in knowledge and skills make it impossible for any one individual doctor to provide the whole span of modern medicine.*

In consequence, there has been a vast growth of specialization with a resultant fragmentation of care, which has been the more pronounced and serious because of the decline in the absolute and relative number of physicians in general practice. This decline, in turn, has been in part due to the fact that general practice has not been generally regarded as a specialty commensurate in status and prestige with other recognized specialties and, until the coming of Medicare and Medicaid, has not offered financial rewards, especially in the poorer neighborhoods, that compare with those reaped by the specialist.

The resulting increase in the use of hospital outpatient departments and even emergency rooms as the point of entry to health services has proved to be no adequate substitute for the family-centered primary physician. This is partly because the hospitals have not been located by reference to the convenience of the populations who need service and partly because these departments too are overly oriented to a concern with specialized and episodic care. What happens to the patient before and after his contact with the hospital appears to be nobody's business.

Nor has this hit-and-miss episodic method of finding entry to the health system solved the problem of redundancy of patient history-taking and the storage and retrieval of essential medical data about patients.

(2) *The rapid advances in medical science and technology lead to a rapid obsolescence of the average practitioner.*

The old policy of licensing for practice once and for all fails to meet the requirements of the present scientific age. In its own defense the community must require additional study or qualifications of those who have been in practice for some specified period and must use its influence and powers to help the practitioner attain acceptable competence. It appears to be generally agreed that a minimum step in this direction would be the requirement of a hospital connection whereby the practitioner would be brought in contact with modern developments of practice and subject to the abrasive stimulus of staff meetings and contact with his peers.

(3) *The necessity to bring together highly skilled professionals,*

4

*expensive and intricate equipment, and pure and applied scientists, and also to provide appropriate patient diagnosis and care has led to an enhancement of the importance and prestige of the hospital.*

But while the hospital has become increasingly attractive to practitioners as the center for research and training and to patients as the locus for the giving and receipt of certain kinds of care, and has tended to become a focal point for the provision of health services *as they are currently delivered,* it is far from certain that the hospital serves, or perhaps even could serve, in this role for the provision of health services *as they should be delivered.* For the voluntary hospitals, answerable to none but their own boards of governors or directors (frequently self-perpetuating and unrepresentative of many of the population groups served) have been in the happy position of being largely free to determine their own role. In particular they have been able to control intake and have tended to concentrate on those episodic complaints that have been the subject of the more spectacular advances in knowledge or skill or which appear to present challenging research or practice opportunities, especially those useful for teaching purposes. They have in large measure refrained from involvement in the total spectrum of community health services, which, it must be emphasized, comprise a range that is far broader than those offered by even the most socially oriented contemporary hospitals. Even in their role as teachers of medical professionals the hospitals have placed emphasis upon the production of specialists in the types of care that are typically provided in a hospital setting. Only recently have there been signs of a revival of interest in community medicine and general practice as areas worthy of specialized study. Perhaps most notable of all has been the relatively slight involvement of the hospital in programs and techniques of prevention.

From this analysis it follows that proposals for reform in the delivery of health services that focus upon the hospital as the vital center around which everything else must be organized and to the needs of which other structures must be adapted in effect put the cart before the horse. The problem today is to reassess and reformulate the role of the hospital as an institution, and of different types or categories of hospitals in the total spectrum of an adequate comprehensive system for the delivery of personal health services.

(4) *The present arrangements governing the distribution of responsibilities for the performance of various functions among agencies and within geographical areas impede the most effective and economical delivery of services.*

For technical reasons some of the new services and techniques call for centralized performance serving a very large geographical and population area. Among these are the operation of a central referral system and of a data bank, the running of a laboratory service for all except the most routine and simple tests, the operation of a city-wide ambulance service or other appropriate forms of transportation and the like. Again, for technical reasons there are differences in the size of the area that can be efficiently and economically served by certain types of skill and equipment. Thus, the service area for open heart surgery, kidney transplants, or cobalt treatments may be very large. On the other hand, the geographical unit for the rendering of primary physicians' services is necessarily quite small. The catchment area of the community hospital is larger, but it is still smaller than the area that can be effectively served by the medical center or teaching hospital.

An orderly system for the delivery of personal health services would be characterized by adjustment of the location of areas of services and of the siting of institutions to the varying market or catchment areas that are indicated by the nature of the service performed. Some central agency, representative of the public interest, must be charged with the responsibility of formulating plans, and suggesting ways and means whereby the rational distribution of institutions and units of service organization might be approximated.

(5) *Effective utilization of the new knowledge, skills, and technical equipment clearly calls for teamwork and a high degree of coordination.*

Among the more obvious of the changes satisfying these requirements are the following:

• Recognition of the fact that solo practice is today outmoded. Group or team practice under public or private auspices is clearly indicated.

• The primary physician who serves as the point of entry to the entire system must be related to the hospital or medical center.

• Isolation of the hospital from the community can no longer be tolerated. Among the more obvious of the areas where the hospital in future should exercise greater or more effective responsibilities are the tasks of assisting practitioners within its catchment area to keep abreast of modern knowledge and practice methodologies, helping in the professional staffing of other local medical institutions such as ambulatory care centers, nursing homes, chronic care facilities and the like, and above all functioning as a service resource for the variety of primary practitioners and their patients in its area.

• There is urgent need for the assignment, to some central authority representative of the public interest, of responsibility for assessing the effectiveness of the system as a whole in providing appropriate personal health services. No one part of the present complex of health agencies, institutions, and professional practitioners can be entrusted with this task. All would bring to it bureaucratic rigidities, professional myopias, and vested interests. Such an organization might or might not be charged with the duty of setting objectives, but it would have the duty of periodically reporting on the extent to which goals were attained and on the existence of gaps and inadequacies, and with making proposals for the remedying of observed inadequacies or inefficiencies. Of necessity it would have to be equipped with a research staff of high caliber and creativity.

(6) *Modern scientific medicine is very costly.*

The period of training for professional personnel is lengthening. The supporting equipment that is regarded as minimal is very costly. The volume of tests called for in a complete diagnosis appears to be growing. Public opinion no longer tolerates the staffing of hospitals with non-professional personnel receiving sweated wages.

In consequence the proportion of gross national product devoted to the health services is steadily rising. Attention must increasingly be directed to ensuring that there is economy in the use of all resources devoted to the provision of health services. This means:

● Assurance that no unnecessary institutional facilities shall be created or, if existing, be allowed to continue.

● The extent and location of highly specialized equipment and specialized procedures must be determined by the size of the service area which can effectively utilize them rather than by the desires of any given institution to be in a position to supply them.

● Expensively trained personnel should be utilized only for procedures necessitating this degree of training and experience. In particular, much more use must be made of the allied health professionals and of nonprofessional workers (in the latter case under professional supervision) and efforts must be directed to training and utilizing available health personnel whose potential now too often goes to waste because of the lack of any effective ladder for advancement. It is obvious, too, that the potentials of automation should be exploited to the full.

● Greater attention must be paid to prevention and to the better health education of people. Desirable in themselves, these objectives will become ever more appealing as the costs of treatment and care continue to rise.

# The Financial Revolution

It is stating a truism to observe that the use of private (commercial and nonprofit) and public (Medicare) insurance, together with Medicaid, has revolutionized the financing of personal health services. Not all of the features of this revolution, however, will necessarily ease the nation's task in developing a more rational and effective health system, even though the new financial arrangements make certain kinds of organizational and structural changes even more imperative.

The implication to which most prominence is given is the expectation that vast new moneys will be available which will enable communities to improve the quality of care and to provide more adequately for meeting health needs. Admittedly both Medicare and Medicaid will make a larger total of funds available to the health system as a whole. This is not merely because the federal government will be paying for or sharing in the costs of certain types of care which were previously a personal, a state, or a state and city responsibility, but also because the federal government has adopted a policy of reimbursing for the "customary and usual charges" of practitioners and for the "reasonable costs," including an allowance for depreciation and obsolescence, in the case of institutions.

But these very policies limit the extent to which communities can use these funds to purchase more or better care. A sizable fraction of the new money must go to increasing the incomes of the providers of care who are now no longer expected to subsidize the government by rendering services below market cost. Only to the extent that higher payments automatically improve the quality of service or to the extent that with more generous "bait" communities can bargain for higher standards of care or greater conformity with policies in the public interest, will these new funds prove to be an additional weapon in their hands for the improvement of the delivery of health services.

Even the use of the new funds as a bargaining weapon to secure certain ends is limited by the fact that their administration is subject to standards and controls laid down by the federal and state governments. Thus, efforts of the New York City Administrator to require certain standards of physicians desiring to participate in Medicaid were nullified by action on the part of the State Health Department (often more sensitive to the views of the organized medical establishment than is the city).

There are also real limits to the extent to which communities can, without securing state approval, use Medicaid money to influence the organization and delivery of health services. Federal law requires that there be a single state agency responsible to it for the expenditure of funds under Title XIX and for the administration of the program, though the latter may be delegated to subordinate political subdivisions operating under state supervision. And it is the federal government which requires that the determination of financial eligibility for Medicaid shall be carried out by the welfare department.

It must also be recalled that some part of the "new money" will be utilized to reimburse local expenditures on behalf of eligible people who have been given claims to free or partly free medical service under the definition of financial eligibility adopted by the state.

That substantial additional funds will flow into the health services system is, however, undeniable. This, plus the fact that the funds come from public sources, will intensify the necessity for policy and organizational changes.

• The new financial situation involves the providers of care in negotiations with large-scale purchasers both private (Blue Cross and Blue Shield as well as commercial insurance companies) and public (the administrators of Medicare and Medicaid). Prices paid will no longer be determined by a largely uncontrolled competitive market, but increasingly by a collective bargaining process in which a variety of interests, considerations, and pressures will play a role. Because of the enhanced visibility of the health bill in which rising prices charged by suppliers will be reflected in higher premiums or taxes, there will be renewed pressure on those who represent the interests of the consumer and purchaser to pay diligent attention to the appropriateness of the prices charged and the reasonableness of the operational costs on which they are allegedly based and to assure that the public is getting value for money. Accountability, both fiscal and performance, will assume new importance and much new research will be called for to develop policies and techniques for testing performance, quality, and benefit in an area where definition and measurement of "product" are notoriously difficult. Inevitably, in this context, those who administer the growing public share of the medical bill will find themselves forced to consider the effect on costs of the way in which health services are organized and administered. To the extent that the present disorderly fragmentation and multiple sponsorship (public, voluntary, and proprietary hospitals and private practitioners) lead to wasteful use of resources both institutional and professional, the new financial arrangements are likely to strengthen the forces working for a more rational organization of personal health services.

Even here, however, the fact that localities share responsibility with the federal and state governments, whose policies prevail, will limit the use which they might otherwise make of their bargaining power with the providers of service to influence the way in which health services are rendered and remunerated. Levels of remuneration will inevitably be influenced, if not effectively determined, by the prices paid by the federal government in connection with the Medicare program.

Use of the Medicaid funds to encourage group practice or prepayment for the purchase of comprehensive care is rendered more difficult by the federal policies adopted under Medicare which in effect leave it to the medical practitioner to decide how he is to be paid. These policies have effectively perpetuated the fee-for-service system, on an item-by-item basis, as the normal method of paying for medical care. It seems likely that systems of prepaid comprehensive care undertaken by groups of physicians will have to be introduced through the public financing of demonstration projects which will presumably "sell" themselves by superior performance in competition with solo practice on an item-by-item, fee-for-service basis.

• A second consequence of the new financial arrangements is that henceforth an ever larger proportion of the recipients of health care will be persons for whom the whole "reasonable" costs of care will be paid for by third parties, and increasingly by government agencies. This will sharply reduce the supply of "charity patients" and thus of the human "teaching material" so necessary for the training of medical personnel and for research. Two solutions would seem to be indicated. On the one hand, efforts should be made to increase the supply of other teaching "bodies" such as dogs and monkeys, which, while expensive to produce and utilize, might effectively fill part of the gap. The other is to press for a policy of utilizing all patients, both public and private, for research and teaching purposes. This would undoubtedly be as shocking to some as the present policy of reliance upon charity patients has been to others. But it could at least be defended on the grounds of democratic treatment and by the consideration that today only relatively few patients pay anything like 100 per cent of the costs of medical care in hospitals from their own pockets.

• A third consequence of the new financial arrangements will be of profound consequence to cities such as New York with its existing systems of voluntary and municipal control and operation of hospitals. For the fact that an increasing number of patients treated in voluntary hospitals will be paid for by public funds will further blur the distinction between what is "voluntary" and what is "public."

In fact, of course, for many years, the so-called voluntary hospital has not been purely, or even predominantly, "voluntary," if by this is meant "supported by philanthropic contributions and fees from private patients." The voluntary hospital of today would be incapable of operating without support from the public sector. This support is not merely financial, although this is highly important, taking the form of tax-privileges allowed taxpayers' contributions to the support of the hospital, tax freedom for property owned or occupied by the hospital, financial aid for construction costs and capital needs as well as the ever-growing grants for research, mainly from the federal government. Equally important is the symbiotic relationship of the voluntary hospitals to the public system. On the one hand government, by financing the supply of charity patients and by operating public hospitals for the poor, has provided the medical schools and voluntary teaching hospitals with badly needed teaching and research material. On the other hand, the existence of the public system has served as a screen to protect the voluntary hospital system as a whole (there are obvious exceptions) from the public criticism that would otherwise have been directed at (1) its operation of a highly selective admission system which reflects neither any rational division of labor among the various hospitals nor concern for the patient group as a whole but is determined primarily by the institutions' needs as research and teaching agencies, (2) its lack of concern with what happens to the patient once he leaves the hospital premises, i.e., an indifference to, or lack of involvement with, the community's health infrastructure, and (3) the failure of the voluntary system to give leadership in the realm of prevention.

In some respects the public and the voluntary hospital systems are in a competitive relationship. In the present state of shortage of trained personnel and of competing demands on limited resources for buildings, equipment, and the like, the voluntary system, answerable only to its own trustees and governed primarily by what is best for the individual hospital as a research and teaching institution, can outcompete the public sector for manpower and can divert resources to the construction of unnecessary facilities.

In view of all these circumstances, the fact that the taxpayer will be financing a growing volume of health service (in some cases over half the income of the "voluntary" institution may be tax money) is perhaps only the final evidence needed to demonstrate that there can no longer be such an entity as a purely "voluntary" hospital system. The voluntary hospital today is a public—or more accurately, a social—utility. As such, it must be more responsive to the coordinated health needs of the community as a whole and held accountable for performance as part of an integrated system for the delivery of health services.

11

Determination of the appropriate role of the existing voluntary hospitals in the complex of health services and assurance that they do indeed undertake, in partnership with the public authorities, the responsibilities indicated by the wider public interest, will be no simple task. For the more important hospitals today have dual responsibilities. On the one hand the hospital performs the vital function of a research and teaching agency with all that this implies for the raising of standards and dissemination of advances in medical science and technology. On the other hand, it is also a provider of personal health services, and an appropriate compromise between the two roles will not be easy to find. Furthermore, it should be noted that should some existing municipal hospitals be improved and equipped to perform research and teaching roles they, too, will face the same dilemma. It is the function, not the sponsorship, that creates the problem.

It is also important to note that the requirement that the hospital of tomorrow be more responsive to the coordinated health needs of the community as a whole does not necessarily imply that all aspects of the functioning of the institution should be subject to governmental fiat and control. The task of the future is to determine which functions in relation to the delivery of personal health services must necessarily be undertaken by a major teaching and research institution and are of such vital importance that their performance cannot be left solely to the decision of the individual institution.

Assurance that the hospitals perform the roles indicated by the public interest can be obtained in a variety of ways. In some cases financial incentives will be sufficient. In others, discussion and negotiation between the leadership of the hospitals and the representatives of the taxpayers will lead to changes in policy as dictated by the public interest. In yet others, regulation and compulsion may be essential. It has, for example, long been accepted that the public interest demands that government have the power to license hospitals. More recently, governmental controls have been invoked in some states to regulate the investment of capital resources in hospital construction and costly equipment.

But whatever the specific functions of the hospital deemed to be charged with a public interest, and whatever the mechanisms adopted to assure their performance, the fact remains that the modern hospital is a social utility and is accountable to the community for the use it makes of the resources that the community entrusts to it.

12

# 2

# The Current
# Delivery System

The health services system is one of the nation's largest industries. In fiscal 1970 America spent over $67 billion (or 7% of the gross national product) on all health services and $58 billion (or 6% of the gross national product) on personal health services alone. In 1965 medical care and related health services ranked sixth in personal consumption expenditures, exceeded only by food, housing, household operation, transportation, and clothing. Furthermore, health expenditures, whether measured in dollar amounts or as a percentage of GNP, have shown a steady upward trend that has been especially pronounced since 1965. The industry currently employs about 2.5 million workers distributed over some forty major job classifications requiring some specific medical training.

## The Nature of the Delivery System

The goods and services made available by the health and medical care system involve the participation of a variety of organizations and individuals. Some of these provide services directly while others carry out related functions such as financing the purchase of services, planning, regulation, resource development, and the like. Some are profit-making. Some are nonprofit organizations governed mainly by the providers. To a much smaller extent, some are nonprofit organizations formed by or operated in the interests of consumers. Finally to an increasing degree governments, federal, state, and local, are involved in the health service system.

### The Private Sector
*Profit-making sector.* The profit-oriented producers include both

Reprinted with permission of the National Association of Social Workers, from the Encyclopedia of Social Work. New York, 1971.

small- and large-scale operators. What has frequently been termed a "cottage industry" is typical of about two thirds of practicing general practitioners and specialists and of most dentists. These suppliers of care function independently, or at best in small partnerships. (Of 4,287 group practices in 1966, half consisted of from three to five members and only 1,375 were general service groups, the remainder being single-specialty partnerships.) They practice in their own small workshops, using such capital equipment as they can afford, and sell their product on a piecework basis to such customers as come their way.

The majority of physicians are in specialist practice. In 1967 there were only 69,000 general practitioners among the 280,000 active physicians. Physicians generally are unevenly distributed about the country, with a greater density in the richer states and the metropolitan areas and a shortage in rural areas and inner-city ghettos.

The majority of physicians are members of the American Medical Association (AMA) although Negroes, who have often been excluded from the AMA, have formed the National Medical Association, and a group of doctors who regard the AMA as illiberal and obstructive of change have formed the Physicians' Forum. Like other professional organizations, the AMA is concerned with maintenance of professional standards, formulation and enforcement of professional ethics, and similar activities directed toward the advancement of medicine and the protection of the interests of its practitioners. In addition, the AMA has actively concerned itself with arrangements for the delivery of health services and their organization and financing. At one time it opposed any form of insurance, public or private. More recently its opposition has been directed to public or social insurance, which until 1965 it fought successfully through political influence and extensive and costly publicity campaigns.

Although the political influence of the AMA has declined markedly since 1965, its continuing advocacy of voluntary, rather than compulsory, insurance, its opposition to any departure from a fee-for-service method of remuneration of practitioners, and its strong preference for solo as against group practice continue to be obstacles in the way of reform of the delivery system.

Medical professionals form the central core of the health services delivery system and control the treatment of the individual patient. They are buttressed, especially if practicing in hospitals, by an ever-growing array of nurses, technical specialists, laboratory technicians, and other paramedical personnel.

Relatively small-scale production for profit is also characteristic of some 850 proprietary short-term hospitals, of much of the retailing of drugs, of the typical nursing home (of which there were some 20,000 in 1966), and of the 700 small drug manufacturing companies who produce only 5% of all prescription drugs.

Among the most important of the large-scale profit-seeking providers are the 136 member companies of the Pharmaceutical Manufacturers Association, who produce 95% of the nation's annual $5 billion drug output. These firms produce and sell both brand name and generic name products; some seventy of them conduct essentially all of the industry's research and control the overwhelming majority of the drug patents. They compete vigorously, mainly on the basis of innovation and quality rather than price, and in general are characterized by high rates of profit. Knowledge of available drugs and sales are promoted by advertising and visits by some twenty thousand "detail men" who visit physicians, hospitals, and pharmacists, and by extensive use of free samples.

In recent years large-scale production has tended to characterize the output of what may be termed "medical hardware" and technical equipment through the formation of mergers, conglomerates, and the entry into these lines of production of large firms who also produce other products.

A very important role in the health services delivery system is played by the large private profit-seeking insurance companies. As the carriers of some $7 billion of private health insurance with a gross enrollment of over 193 million persons representing (according to various estimates) between 152 million and 169 million different persons, they influence the delivery system by writing policies in which the costs of all or part of specified benefits are reimbursed. Such policies enable the private company to control its cost commitments but they contribute to the fragmentation of services that is currently so often criticized. Since 1965 some commercial insurance companies have also served as financial intermediaries in connection with Medicare for both parts of the program. As such they administer the payments made to hospitals and other qualifying institutions and to physicians, subject to broad guiding principles laid down by the Social Security Administration.

*The nonprofit sector.* Nonprofit operation characterizes the second major private group involved in the organization, delivery, and financing of health services. Nonprofit hospitalization insurance is dominated by seventy-five Blue Cross schemes with a membership of some 68 million which are affiliated in a national organization, the Blue Cross Association. Medically organized schemes, the so-called Blue Shield insurance systems of which there are seventy-three with a

15

membership of 60 million, provide some coverage against the costs of physicians' services. The Blue Cross-Blue Shield plans have in recent years been losing business to the commercial plans. Although originally stressing service benefits, rather than indemnification of some fraction of the costs of specific services, and the setting of community rates, they have been forced by this competition increasingly to resort to indemnity payments and experience rating. It is noteworthy that both Blue Shield and Blue Cross are organized by, and administered in the interests of, the providers of the services that they purchase.

Prominent among the group of nonprofit providers are the voluntary hospitals; there were 3,440 in 1966 and they can best be described as independent fiefdoms. Typically they are short-term general hospitals but many are teaching hospitals and some are operated as integral parts of university-affiliated medical centers. They enjoy tax-exempt status presumably because they receive support from philanthropic funds (which in turn are tax deductible) and because they provide services on a charitable basis. Indeed, until a ruling of the Internal Revenue Service in October 1969, charitable service was required to secure tax exemption. To an increasing degree, however, the voluntary hospital today relies heavily on public funds, in the form of grants for research (somewhat flexibly defined), loans and grants for construction, and reimbursement of all or part of the costs of services provided to specified categories of patients.

The voluntary hospitals are governed by boards of directors or trustees whose composition reflects the earlier dependence of the hospital on philanthropic support. The members tend to represent the more affluent and influential people in the community; representation by the mass of consumers of the hospital's services or by governmental authorities providing sizable financial support is rare or nonexistent. These governing bodies are responsible only to themselves, apart from conformity with legal or professional requirements for accreditation or licensing. It is this body that determines what shall be the role of the hospital, what services it will offer, and which population groups it will serve.

Technical and scientific developments have conspired to place the hospital, voluntary or public, in a key position in the health care system. It makes possible the provision of the increasingly costly and elaborate equipment and skilled supporting services so necessary to the efficient practice of modern medicine. It offers a convenient facility for its affiliated physicians and raises standards of practice by providing opportunity for peer contact, consultation, and criticism. The medical schools use the hospital as a laboratory for both teaching and research

16

and have been responsible for much of the spectacular improvement in scientific medicine and medical techniques.

The hospitals typically concentrate on episodic care and on the so-called horizontal patient who occupies a bed. Most hospitals operate outpatient departments and emergency rooms which have become increasingly important as the growing shortage of family physicians has caused more people (notably the poor) to use these facilities as substitutes. But ambulatory care has not been accorded the interest or the prestige assigned to care of the bedpatient. Nor have most hospitals been deeply involved in the operation and development of community health services or given much leadership in preventive health programs.

Another, less frequently found group of nonprofit organizations delivering health services are the prepaid group practice plans. For what is actually or in effect a capitation fee, they undertake to provide the full spectrum of services needed by the subscriber through organized multispecialty physician groups linked with hospitals and other services. The most noteworthy of these plans are the Kaiser Permanente Medical Care Programs, which originated on the West Coast and are now spreading to other states. These have grown from 30,000 members in 1946 to around 2 million in 1970. And the Health Insurance Plan of Greater New York has a current membership of approximately 800,000.

Programs of this type have grown but slowly, however. In total only 3% of the clinical visits in the country are made by ambulatory patients to prepaid group practices. There are many reasons for the slow growth of systems that would seem to offer a method of insuring comprehensive and continuous care. In some states legal barriers to this form of practice exist. In others the opposition of organized medicine has discouraged physicians from participating. The problem of obtaining a connection with, and control over the policies of, essential hospitals, or funds to purchase or construct a hospital, has been formidable. With voluntary enrollment there is always the problem of insuring funds to finance a newly initiated system until enrollment is large enough to support the range of services and facilities that must be available from the outset.

Nonprofit comprehensive health service organizations formed or managed by consumers are even less frequently found. Some of the collectively bargained health insurance plans (which in total covered some 4.7 million persons in 1968) were thus organized, but recently many self-insured groups have taken out coverage with Blue Cross-Blue Shield or commercial insurance companies. A relatively small program of comprehensive health services organized in the interests of the

17

consumers has been operated under the Economic Opportunity Act of 1966. Building on experiments undertaken in 1965, funds became available to support neighborhood health centers providing accessible and dignified personal health services to low-income families with maximum feasible participation of the poor. Some forty-eight such centers have been developed, usually as part of the community action program. Generally the operating agents are health departments, medical schools, hospitals, or group practice organizations. The plans aim to offer a complete range of health services, make arrangements with other organizations for specialized services when necessary, and to emphasize outreach and convenience of access. Eligibility for these services is usually limited to the poor or near-poor.

### The Role of Government

Until recently the involvement of government, and especially the federal government, in the health services complex was relatively slight, at least as compared with the situation in other countries. But during the 1960s a flood of legislation greatly extended the range of government's health responsibilities and by 1970 governmental participation took a number of forms.

*Supportive services.* Governments, mainly state and local, are responsible for protective and supportive environmental health services, a function that they have long had. These services include the traditional "public health" concern with water supplies, sewage disposal, and the like, and with disease control or prevention programs. Although their activities in these areas in the past have achieved considerable success, they are now criticized for failure to control environmental hazards, including air and water pollution, radiation hazards, contamination of foodstuffs by chemicals, and the like. It remains to be seen whether the creation of a new agency in the federal Public Health Service, the Consumer Protection and Environmental Health Service, following the passage of the Clean Air Act of 1963 and the Air Quality Act of 1967, will foster more aggressive leadership in this area.

*Licensing.* Governments are concerned with assuring the quality of health services. Licensing of physicians is mandatory in all states. The object of the laws, which are usually administered through state boards of medical examiners, is to protect the public against incompetence, quackery, or unscientific principles in medical practice. Licensing laws covering allied and auxiliary health personnel have usually been "friendly" regulations enacted with the cooperation of the professions and occupations involved. They aim to protect both the regulated personnel and the public from unqualified and unethical practitioners and, because the license is limited to a particular segment of the health services, they involve a determination of the services that a licensee may not legally perform.

Most states provide for the licensing of hospitals and, to a lesser degree, other medical facilities. Under the provisions of Medicare and Medicaid, state agencies are required to assure that participating hospitals and other institutions comply with broad federal standards. But for the voluntary program of the Joint Commission on the Accreditation of Hospitals, there is no other systematic evaluation of the quality of care given in hospitals.

The federal Food and Drug Administration has long been responsible for monitoring the quality, effectiveness, and safety of drugs and has extensive responsibilities in regard to the purity, quality, and packaging of food products.

*Personnel and facilities.* Governments have become increasingly active in regard to the supply of personnel and facilities. The Health Professions Educational Assistance Act of 1963, with amendments in 1965, aims to increase the supply of health professionals, especially physicians. Federal grants are provided to assist in the construction and operation of facilities for the training of health professionals and to give some financial assistance to students. The Nurse Training Act of 1964, the Allied Health Professions Act, and part of the Manpower Development and Training Act aim to increase the supply of trained nurses and other auxiliary personnel. Over a period of twenty years, grants and technical assistance from the National Institutes of Mental Health have trained over thirty-four thousand mental health professionals. Training programs of more limited scope are also supported by the Children's Bureau and the Office of Economic Opportunity.

Starting in 1946, the Hill-Burton (now Hill-Harris) Act had by 1968 approved 9,549 federally aided hospital construction projects at a total cost of $10 billion, of which the federal share was $3.1 billion. Originally the main thrust of the Hill-Burton program was in the rural areas. More recently some federal aid has become available for the construction of nursing homes, and it is currently being suggested that the program be extended to ambulatory facilities and modernization of urban hospitals.

*Individual services.* Governments are to some extent involved in the direct provision of health services to individuals. The states have long operated facilities for the custody and/or treatment of persons suffering from tuberculosis or mental illness. In some areas there are public clinics for the treatment of venereal disease. A number of communities, of which New York City is perhaps the most noteworthy, operate municipal hospitals for the care of the needy or medically indigent. The federal government provides medical care to seamen, members of the armed forces, veterans, Indians, and important members and officials of the government.

State and local maternal and child health programs under the Child Health Act of 1967 (the old Title V of the Social Security Act shorn of the child welfare services) were providing maternity clinic services to 366,400 expectant mothers in 1967, while some 73,000 received inpatient hospital care. Over 1.5 million children were seen in well-child conferences and many more school children were screened although by no means always treated for general physical conditions and visual, hearing, or dental defects. Finally state and local authorities provide public health nurses who work in the homes and elsewhere in the community, and, much more rarely, homemaker services.

*Financial aid.* Governments have become increasingly involved in programs directed toward meeting the costs of personal health services. Between 1950 and 1969 the proportion of personal health care expenditures carried by government rose from 19.9% to 35.6%, of which two-thirds came from the federal government.

All the states and the federal government have enacted workmen's compensation laws that cover some or all of the costs of medical care provided to workers who are injured or who contract diseases in the course of their employment. The state laws vary widely in the proportion of workers covered and the illnesses and the range of medical benefits that are included.

The federal government also shares in the cost of health insurance for its own employees (the Federal Employees Health Benefits Program) and finances a program of health care for the dependents of members of the armed forces (the original Medicare program now known as CHAMPUS).

State and/or local public assistance authorities have long financed health services of varying scope and quality for public assistance recipients. Expenditures for this purpose greatly increased after 1950 when, under the Social Security Act amendments, the federal government began to share in the costs of vendor payments for medical care of the federally assisted categories. The Kerr-Mills Act of 1960 broadened the coverage of this financial aid by including also the medically indigent aged and by liberalizing some eligibility conditions. The Medicaid program, initiated by Title XIX of the Social Security Amendments of 1965, aimed to extend the program to all medically indigent and especially children so that by a foreseeable date (originally 1975 but subsequently postponed to 1977) no person would be denied adequate health care because of financial incapacity.

By 1970 all states except Alaska and Arizona had Medicaid plans in operation or expected to commence them shortly. The scope of the services provided and the range of persons covered (largely determined by the income limits set by the state) varied greatly among the states. Most programs are administered by welfare departments which have traditionally paid little attention to quality of care or the circumstances accompanying its receipt. Even so, the cost of this program has greatly exceeded congressional expectations. By 1965 total medical vendor payments amounted to $1.3 billion or about 130% above the 1960 level. By January, 1968, when only thirty-seven states had adopted the Medicaid program, annual federal costs were estimated at $3.4 billion. State and local expenditures amounted in 1968 to $1.9 billion. As compared with 1965 they rose from less than one-third to almost one-half of total welfare expenditures (less administrative costs). Federal amendments adopted in 1967 and 1969 aimed at keeping total costs under control by sharply lowering the income limit for the medically indigent in whose costs the federal government would share, by reducing the minimum package of health services that any participating state was required to offer, and by postponing the date by which comprehensive services would be available to all regardless of ability to pay. One third of the states adopting plans in 1966 or 1967 initiated or planned for cutbacks in their scope or coverage. Even so the 1970 budget estimated federal Medicaid costs at $3.1 billion.

Governmental involvement in the health services system was greatly expanded by the enactment of Medicare (Title XVIII of the Social Security Amendments of 1965), which instituted a system of health insurance for the aged. In fiscal 1970 expenditures for this program amounted to $7.1 billion, or 42% of all federal health outlays. A distinction was made between hospital care and related extended care and home health care, which are provided for under Title XVIIIA, and the services of physicians, provided for under Title XVIIIB. For Title XVIIIA benefits insurance is compulsory and paid-up by age 65, and, except for the blanketing-in of aged persons not previously insured under the Social Security Act, is financed entirely by wage and payroll taxes. Title XVIIIB insurance is voluntary, with the federal government contributing 50% of the premium, and is not paid up. Both parts are essentially reimbursement systems, covering only specified types or amounts of health services on an item-by-item basis, and are accompanied by deductibles, copayments and coinsurance. While subject to the overriding administrative authority of the Secretary of Health, Education and Welfare acting through the Social Security Administration, which also maintains eligibility records, the day-to-day administration of payments to providers is in the hands of fiscal intermediaries such as Blue Cross or Blue Shield or private insurance companies. A small number of providers deal directly with the federal administration.

*Research programs.* Another governmental activity bearing on the health services system is support of research, expenditures for which have increased sharply in recent years, from $72.9 million in fiscal 1950 to $1.69 billion in fiscal 1970, all but $73 million of which came from the federal government. During the same period private expenditures for medical research increased from $37 million to $195 million. Some of the supported research is undertaken directly by the federal government through various divisions of the Public Health Service, such as the National Institutes of Health, the National Center for Health Services and Development, and the National Center for Health Statistics. But much federally supported research takes the form of grants and research contracts to state and local agencies, private institutions, universities, hospitals, and individuals outside the federal government. Other components of the Department of Health, Education and Welfare, such as the Children's Bureau, also administer research funds.

It will be noted from this account of governmental activities in the field of the health services that there has been great reluctance on the part of governments to become involved with the health services delivery system itself. Governments have in general accepted the status quo and refrained from requiring any particular organizational structure or any particular method of supplying service or of remunerating providers. Indeed the preamble to Title XVIII states specifically that "nothing in this section shall be construed to authorize any federal officer or employee to exercise any supervision or control over the manner in which medical services are provided . . . or to exercise any supervision or control over the administration of any institution, agency or person."

Nor have governments until recently been directly concerned with the efficiency of providers and the system of which they are a part. Even the research undertaken or financed by government has concentrated on clinical medicine to the neglect of research into organization and the delivery system.

In many respects governmental programs have tended to perpetuate the existing fragmentation of service. They have been developed on the basis of defined categories of persons (the old, the young, the poor, the veteran, and so on) or types of disease or treatment or kinds of institutions, and they have adopted a reimbursement rather than a service approach and have supported the fee-for-service method of remuneration. It seems likely that this deference to the established delivery system and to the convenience and preferences of providers will be modified in the future, if only because of government's concern about rising costs. A number of the proposals for national health insurance introduced into the Congress in 1970 attempted to use the financial leverage of the insurance funds to promote a more rational delivery system.

Meanwhile, a number of governmental programs were beginning to grapple with the delivery problem. As part of its responsibility to "promote the mental health of the people of the United States," the National Institutes of Mental Health fostered the development of community mental health centers by grants for construction and/or staffing. One of the institute's major goals is the modernization of the nation's outdated system for delivery of mental health services. Thirty-three states now have community mental health service acts providing state aid for local services. Nevertheless, some critics deplore the concentration on mental health as serving still further to perpetuate fragmentation of service.

By 1968, fifty-three maternity and infant care projects were providing comprehensive care to mothers and infants from low-income families under the auspices of the Children's Bureau. Efforts were made in these projects to coordinate all available community services, including transportation, additional foods, homemaker services, and by the use of mobile clinics, extended hours of operation, and more publicity to bring the services within reach of those who could profit from them.

*Regional planning.* Two recent federal enactments have provided encouragement for state and regional planning. The Regional Medical Programs Act of 1965 as amended offered planning grants and operational funds to regional organizations with the object of improving the quality and the availability of diagnosis and care in heart disease, cancer, stroke, and related diseases, thereby reducing the time lag, so often the subject of complaint, between new knowledge and its translation into practice. By the end of 1968, fifty-five regional medical programs covering the entire United States were in receipt of federal funds.

This concentration on specific diseases is deplored in many medical circles as further encouraging fragmentation. Not wholly clear, moreover, is the relation of those bodies to the planning authorities whose encouragement is the object of the Comprehensive Health Planning and Public Health Services Amendments of 1966 (PL 89-749), sometimes known as the Partnership for Health Act. This act provides formula grants to states for comprehensive health planning, project grants for comprehensive areawide, or local comprehensive, planning, project grants for training studies and demonstrations, formula grants for health services, and project grants for health services development. By mid-1968 all the states, the District of Columbia, and four territories were actively participating in the planning program.

The federal administration also renewed emphasis on problems related to the health services delivery system. In 1968 the National Center for Health Services Research and Development was created to provide coordination and leadership for all research and development activities aimed at improving the quality and delivery of health services. Through contracts it conducts and supports research, development, demonstration, and training projects concerned with the organization, utilization, distribution, quality, and financing of health services, and facilities. Under Section 314 of the Public Health Service Act federally financed support for neighborhood health centers and certain systems of prepaid group practice is available.

At the federal level, progress toward a more rational delivery system is impeded by the dispersion of authority in health matters among many agencies. At least twenty-four different agencies are involved, although the Departments of Health, Education and Welfare, of Defense, and the Veterans Administration account for about 95% of federal health expenditures. Coordination of policy among these agencies is poor. Even within the highly important Department of Health, Education and Welfare, health responsibilities are spread among a number of largely autonomous subdepartments subject only to the authority of an assistant secretary for health and scientific affairs, with limited prestige and staff. Indeed, the Medicare and Medicaid programs are outside his jurisdiction. In consequence, not only is there a lack of clear purpose and system of priorities (with, on occasion, one department implementing policies that run counter to those of another) but when federal involvement takes the form of grants for specific purposes, there is also confusion among grant applicants and much unnecessary "shopping around" and the tailoring of proposals and projects to meet the believed requirements or interests of various departments.

Several proposals have been made to end this dispersion of federal authority. They include removal of health functions from some agencies, increasing the authority and power of the Department of Health, Education and Welfare's chief health official by elevating him to the status of undersecretary, and increasing his staff, and the creation of a Federal Council of Health Advisers corresponding to the Council of Economic Advisers to monitor performance, identify priority needs, and formulate recommendations for national health policy.

## Evaluation of the Delivery System

The variety and large number of institutions and individuals involved in the delivery of health and medical services suggest that there may be justification for the frequently expressed view that existing arrangements must be characterized as a "nonsystem" rather than a system of health care delivery. Its functioning is indeed increasingly being called into question.

*The market model.* Until recently health services have been treated as if they were similar to all other commodities bought and sold on the open market. In this system of economic organization competing producers offer their wares to consumers who buy or reject them on the basis of the quality and price of the product. The high-priced producer or the one who fails accurately to forecast what consumers want makes no profit and is driven from the market. Thus the consumer determines what shall be produced. At the same time the market system ensures economy in the use of resources, because the inefficient producer who uses resources uneconomically will have high costs, be unable to meet the prices of his more efficient competitors, and sooner or later will disappear from the scene.

This market model is, however, peculiarly inappropriate for several reasons when applied to the health and medical care services.

(1) The quality of the product is difficult for the consumer to judge effectively, and this difficulty has increased as medicine has become more highly technical and scientific. Consumers find it increasingly difficult to appraise the competence of primary physicians or specialists, the usefulness of diagnostic tests, the quality of hospital care, or the efficacy of drugs. In addition much of medical care, especially the most

25

costly, is required on a one-time basis. Thus, unlike the consumer of commodities meeting recurrent needs, the consumer of health and medical care services, even assuming he recovers, cannot profit by his past experience and change his selection of suppliers accordingly.

(2) The consumer has in practice only a limited range of choice. His selection is essentially restricted to a primary physician or, in case of self-diagnosis, a specialist. Thereafter his purchase of the needed spectrum of health services is in the hands of his physician who advises about, and usually arranges for, subsequent diagnostic tests, specialist services, needed drugs and, when necessary, entry into hospital.

(3) At the time he needs medical care the consumer is frequently in no position to shop around or to bargain about, or even question, price.

(4) Price competition, except perhaps in the retail sale of drugs, scarcely exists in the medical care industry. Physicians neither advertise their prices nor vaunt their own wares and decry those of their competitors. The same applies to institutional care. This absence of price competition among providers not only deprives the consumer of the possibility of making selections on the basis of price but, perhaps even more importantly, removes the pressure for elimination of the high-cost producer that exists in the economic market.

Thus the extent to which the health services delivery system meets the needs of consumers and does so at minimal cost cannot be judged by ordinary market criteria. Yet alternative criteria are not easy to apply. The product of the industry is difficult to define and measure. Presumably the end product is good health, but there is little or no agreement on its components. In global terms, efforts to measure the health status of the American population by the use of such indices as infant and maternal death rates, death rates among men aged 40-65, or morbidity data suggest that the performance of the industry leaves much to be desired, at least as compared with the situation in many other countries. Health is affected, however, not only by the efficiency of the specific health service providers but also by a host of other conditions such as levels of income and standards of living, quality of nutrition or housing, environmental pollution, and the like.

In these circumstances the effectiveness of the health services industry has usually been judged by its ability to meet certain specific needs expressed by consumers. These in brief are for the convenient and continuous availability of appropriate and high quality preventive, diagnostic, curative, and rehabilitative services, rendered in a manner that respects the dignity of the recipient and is technically efficient and economical in the use of the nation's productive resources. By reference to these criteria the nation's "system" for the delivery of health services, in contrast to the generally high reputation of American technical and scientific clinical practice and medical research, must be judged gravely deficient.

Its shortcomings have been documented and reiterated by a long series of investigations, commissions, hearings, conferences, and task forces beginning with the now classic report of the Committee on the Cost of Medical Care in 1932, whose conclusions are still depressingly relevant to the present situation. Among the more important findings of these studies are the following:

*Inability to obtain needed services.* Too many people are unable to secure health services. The present system undoubtedly provides needed health services to the majority, albeit at a rapidly increasing cost and with wide variations in quality. But many millions are unable to obtain the care they need. This inability is attributable in many cases to financial barriers that have become higher as science and technology have raised the standards of what is held to be good medical care and, more especially in recent years, as unit prices have risen sharply.

Voluntary adjustment of fees and charges by providers by reference to the financial status of the patient has proved ineffective. Patients dislike accepting charity from their doctors and most doctors dislike the interposition of financial considerations between themselves and their patients, even when they can recoup themselves by overcharging their wealthy patients, which they cannot always do. Hospitals have found the flow of philanthropic funds inadequate to permit them to give all the free or subsidized care demanded and have increasingly sought and received reimbursement from public welfare authorities.

Efforts to remove the financial barrier through private nonprofit or profit-making insurance have had only limited success. A spectacular growth of private insurance has occurred in the last thirty years, from 12 million persons with some insurance against hospitalization in 1940 to over 193 million in 1968, and from 4 million insured for surgical benefits in 1940 to 177 million in 1968 (some persons carried more than one policy). Yet of the 178 million Americans then under age 65, 24 million (13.5%) had no hospital insurance, 35 million (20.9%) had no surgical insurance, 61 million (34.5%) had no in-hospital medical expense insurance, and 102 million (57.2%) had no insurance for doctors' visits in the home or office. Furthermore, by no means were all services covered. Only 2.9% of the population was covered for dental care and 9.6% for nursing home care, while the percentage covered for prescribed drugs, private duty nursing, and visiting nurse services varied between 39.9% and 45.5%. In addition, deductibles and coinsurance in

27

most policies caused indemnity payments often to fall short of actual charges. Hence, by 1969 private insurance paid for only 37% of all consumers' expenditures for personal health services, which in turn accounted for 63% of total national expenditures for personal health services, the remaining 37% coming from government (35%) and philanthropy (2%).

By 1970 public health insurance, apart from Workmen's Compensation laws to which reference has already been made, applied only to the aged. Its effectiveness in removing the financial barrier was limited by the exclusion from reimbursement of many types of care or treatment, by the existence of deductibles and coinsurance, by the absence of scheduled charges to which physicians must conform, and by price escalation that necessitated the raising of premiums and taxes. In addition, only hospitalization and related institutional care was provided through compulsory paid-up insurance. Insurance against the costs of professional services was voluntary but it was government-subsidized and are not paid-up.

As increasing costs compelled the private insurance carriers, both profit and nonprofit, to raise their premiums or cut down benefits, the fear was widely expressed that private insurance was pricing itself out of the market. Demands increased for the extension of public and subsidized health insurance to groups other than the aged, as well as for more comprehensive service coverage. Numerous health insurance bills were introduced into Congress during 1969 and 1970.

Inability to secure needed health services is attributable not only to financial barriers—it is also due to a shortage or maldistribution of manpower and facilities. Although no unanimity exists as to the precise extent of the manpower shortage, all observers agree on the short- and long-run need for a greatly increased supply of health service personnel—scientists, teachers, practitioners, administrators, and paramedical workers.

Suggestions for overcoming the manpower shortage include greater use of public funds to support construction and operation of various types of educational facilities; financial assistance to trainees; a reassessment of the tasks to be performed by various categories of health personnel with a view to more efficient use of highly trained professionals and greater utilization of auxiliary and paraprofessional workers; development of career ladders to broaden the basis of recruitment; changes in the medical curriculum to shorten the period of training and render it more appropriate to the functions performed by different types of physicians; efforts to increase the productivity of physicians; proposals (notably in the case of nurses) to raise levels of remuneration; and development of a more efficient delivery system that would utilize the existing supply of manpower more effectively.

The geographical maldistribution of medical personnel as evidenced by the underdoctored state of rural areas and urban ghettos has not proved easy to remedy. Standardization of the requirements for licensure so as to remove legal barriers to geographical mobility has been proposed, but it would seem that the most acute problem is not interstate but rather intrastate maldistribution. Suggestions have been made for committed fellowships or for cancellation of some portion of student loans in return for specified periods of employment after graduation in underdoctored areas, but such modest experiments of this kind have yielded little. Nor can it be said that much success has come from efforts to deal with the problem of the functional maldistribution of physicians, namely the trend toward specialized practice.

*Fragmentation of care.* Second only to complaints about the inability of too many people to obtain needed health services is the charge which occurs with increasing frequency that the present health delivery system results in fragmentation of care. What should be an integrated and continuous service is, in fact, paid for and provided in small pieces or separate units of care. With the exception of a small number of prepaid hospital based or connected group-practice plans, no overall institutions exist to ensure that the contributions of this great variety of providers are appropriately meshed so that the individual consumer is assured of comprehensive and continuous care. It is as if the consumer of automobiles (a product that also necessitates the integration of a great variety of products, procedures, and providers) were left to locate the various parts and providers for himself and put them together into something resembling a car.

Even if the individual is fortunate enough to have a family or primary physician, his route through the maze of providers depends on the skill, knowledge, and concern of his doctor. In fact the quality of service provided by practitioners ranges from outstanding to poor. Minimal competence is supposedly assured by the existence of licensing laws. Yet despite the tremendous advances in medical science and technology in recent years, no state attempts to prevent educational obsolescence by requiring evidence of further education or professional growth as a condition for maintaining licensure in good standing. Many physicians in private practice are not affiliated with a hospital. Furthermore, community medicine was until recently almost completely neglected in medical school curricula, and professional interest in the nature of the community's delivery system was minimal.

29

The patient who has to use the outpatient department or the emergency room as his point of entry into the health services stream is even worse off, for he cannot even be sure of seeing the same professional on each consultation. Much care in the hospital's ambulatory facilities is provided by overworked residents and interns and the conditions under which it is available are frequently, if not degrading, at least characterized by little respect for the recipients' dignity or their physical comfort or convenience, and by long waiting periods in unprepossessing premises.

Specialization in medical practice is reflected in specialized clinics, so that a family or even an individual may have to visit several geographically separate clinics, each of which is concerned with one pathological condition or organ.

Nor is needed entry into a hospital automatically assured. Quite apart from the financial barriers, not all physicians have hospital connections. Some teaching and research-oriented hospitals allegedly select patients on the basis of the interest of the case or disease as teaching or research material. Voluntary hospitals have been further charged with showing too little concern about what happens to the patients they do not accept and with failing to give adequate support to the public hospitals that, having to accept all who come, in effect protect the voluntary hospitals from criticism for their selective intake. The result is an increasing divergence between the quality of care given in the two types of institutions. The voluntary hospital can maintain high quality and pleasant amenities because it can limit admissions. With open admission and limited funds, the public hospital must spread its resources thin, with a resulting lowering of the quality of care.

Within the confines of the hospital patients can be assured of continuous care, and to this extent the hospital can be described as one of the few highly integrated systems in the spectrum of health services. But hospitals carefully limit the range of their responsibilities and tend to neglect segments of the health care system in which they might be in a strategic position to exert influence and leadership. Hospitals are accused of being largely unconcerned with the patient once he is in an upright position and has left their doors. They are charged with failing to give adequate support to the development of the auxiliary community health services that are particularly necessary as, with rising hospital costs, efforts are made to discharge patients speedily. Nor have the hospitals been greatly involved in raising the standards of practice of solo practitioners in their catchment areas. Affiliation with a hospital is an effective method of keeping physicians abreast of new developments in medical science and practice and exposing them to the stimulating influence of peer judgment. Although the hospitals can rightly claim that not all local doctors could meet affiliation standards of professional competence, critics assert that the hospitals could do more to bring them up to standard.

The growing tendency to look to the hospital as the crucial unit in the health service delivery system and to criticize it for non-performance stems from the fact that the key problem is held to be one of devising and effectuating appropriate linkages between the various services and suppliers. Given the nature of modern medical knowledge and technology, the hospital is at once one of the most important elements in the delivery system and also the one that is large and powerful enough to take the initiative in improving the present delivery system. Many of the health insurance proposals introduced into Congress in 1970 have included measures in the form of grants, loans, and standards for participation to encourage the development of hospital-based group practice and the assumption of wider responsibilities by the hospitals.

*Uneconomic use of resources.* Another criticism of the current delivery system is that it does not ensure economy in the use of resources devoted to health services. Notably since 1965 public and congressional concern has increased about the sharply mounting costs of health services, which are due to a number of factors:

(1) There appears to be an overinvestment of capital resources in certain types of hospitals, facilities, and equipment. Some hospitals are built or expanded in excess of the need for such facilities in the community. The prestige associated with certain types of medical procedures leads to professional and institutional pressure in hospitals to develop facilities for such expensive procedures as heart transplantation, kidney dialysis, brain surgery, cobalt treatments, and the like to a point where some of these expensive resources and personnel remain underutilized.

Efforts by the community to control unnecessary or poorly located construction and the unnecessary purchase of costly equipment have so far had limited success. The development of state and regional planning agencies, notably under the Partnership for Health legislation, may encourage more sophisticated and widely disseminated evaluation of the health needs and resources of specific communities. But unless these planning agencies are given some authority to require conformity with their plans (and only New York State under the Folsom Act and California have so far taken such power), their influence will remain in doubt. However, many of the proposals for national health insurance or for reform of Medicare and Medicaid introduced into Congress in 1970 and later make some efforts to strengthen the control of these planning bodies. For example, they provide that there will be no federal reimbursement of construction costs unless the proposed investment has been approved by some specified regional, state, or local planning body.

(2) Some share of the increasing proportion of gross national product taken by the health services can be attributed to unnecessary usage of personnel or facilities. All available evidence suggests that, apart perhaps from drugs, overutilization of the health services on the initiative of patients is not generally a major problem. Considerable concern is indeed voiced about underutilization of available services, especially on the part of the poor. Nevertheless, Medicare (and to a more limited degree Medicaid) provides against the believed danger of overutilization by the requirement of deductibles and coinsurance (a policy condemned by many health authorities as likely to discourage early diagnosis and preventive care) and requirements for utilization review in hospitals and extended care facilities.

Much more important is the overuse of that most expensive component in the spectrum of health services, hospital care, which in 1969 accounted for 40% of all spending for health services and supplies. On the one hand, too many patients occupy expensive hospital beds because of the lack of other more appropriate and less costly facilities—nursing homes, extended care facilities, home nursing services, and the like. On the other hand, the system of reimbursement characteristic of private profit and nonprofit health insurance systems finances certain services only if delivered in hospitals. (Even Medicare has not wholly freed itself of this limitation.) Hence some patients occupy hospital beds for purely financial reasons. Concern about overutilization of the hospital led to the inclusion in the Social Security Amendments of 1965 of provision of benefits in extended care facilities and of a requirement for the creation of utilization committees in all participating hospitals. There is some difference of opinion about the effectiveness of this device, however, which necessarily involves peer review.

Control over the use of health services is ultimately in the hands of professionals, especially physicians. While the vast majority of physicians are undoubtedly highly ethical, experience under Medicare and Medicaid suggests that a marginal group has been unable to resist the temptation offered by a fee-for-service reimbursement system to provide, or at least to charge for, unnecessary services. Perhaps of more general concern, especially in view of the professional's fear of malpractice suits, is the encouragement offered by prepaid systems that cover diagnostic tests to overutilize diagnostic facilities and procedures. The absence of central data accumulation and retrieval systems coupled with the fragmentation of care enhances the likelihood of both duplication of tests and nonutilization of the full scope of available data about any given patient.

(3) Inefficient operation of a service adds to costs and wastes resources. Costs, as measured on the basis of bed days, patient days, or patient stays, vary widely among hospitals. Even when allowance is made for differences in treatment and services provided and in local costs of living and wage rates, cost variations remain that can only be attributed to varying degrees of efficiency in individual hospitals. Various investigating bodies have deplored the lack of attention currently paid to the training of hospital administrators. But even if the hospital administrator were to be more suitably trained for his exacting duties, a redefinition of his role vis-à-vis the medical and nursing staffs will be necessary if he is to exercise appropriate authority in running his institution.

Moreover, apart from differences among individual hospitals, there are economies of scale in the form of joint purchasing of supplies, central laundry facilities, centralized food preparation, common data banks, and the like, of which advantage is not adequately taken so long as each hospital functions as an independent entity. Many hospitals, too, are uneconomically small.

(4) Unfortunately the financial arrangements adopted under Medicare and Medicaid, which in effect reimburse each institution on a cost-plus basis, have tended to encourage inefficiency and wasteful use of resources. Every inquiry into the operation of these programs has concluded that there is an imperative need to build financial incentives for efficiency and economy into the reimbursement formula. Some recent health insurance proposals would go so far as to substitute a capitation system for the present item-by-item or cost-plus reimbursement system, and the proposed addition of a Health Maintenance Organization option under Medicare also envisages the expansion of prepaid comprehensive group practice financed from the insurance funds on a capitation basis as a method of providing service more economically.

(5) Wasteful use of resources appears also to characterize the drug-manufacturing industry. The 1969 Task Force on Prescription Drugs found that much of the drug industry's research and development provide only minor contributions to medical progress. The task force complained of the waste of manpower devoted to duplication of essentially identical products and of the clinical facilities needed to test

them.

(6) High costs and wasteful use of resources occur when highly trained personnel perform functions that could be delegated to less expensively trained workers, either acting independently under license or under the supervision of licensed practitioners. Like the social work profession, the medical profession is under strong pressure to reassess the nature of its practice with a view to identifying tasks that could be performed by auxiliary personnel.

(7) The rising costs of the health services reflect not only inefficient or wasteful use of the resources devoted to health care—they are also caused by increases in the unit prices charged by providers. Some part of the rising costs of hospital care is attributable to a long-overdue increase in the salaries and wages of service and paraprofessional personnel. Adoption in the Medicare program of a system of paying physicians on a fee-for-service basis in which the standard of payment is the customary and prevailing charge has in effect permitted physicians to set their own fees. Hitherto private intermediaries who administer the reimbursement system on behalf of the federal government have not been effective in controlling a sharp escalation of charges.

Here again proposals are under consideration for changing the method of remuneration or the terms of the reimbursement formula or for setting legal limits to the extent of cost escalation in any given year. Some authorities, however, doubt whether there is any solution so long as the fee-for-service basis of remuneration is retained. They urge a shift either to salary or capitation. In any case far less attention is paid to reducing costs and ensuring efficiency in respect to medical practitioners than in regard to institutional providers, and public policy in general appears to be more concerned with controlling costs than with assuring a high quality of care or improving the delivery systems.

## REFERENCES

Burns, E.M.: Some major policy decisions facing the United States in the financing and organization of health care. *New Directions in Public Policy for Health Care.* New York, New York Academy of Medicine, December 1966, 1072-1088.

Closing the gaps in the availability and accessibility of health services. *Bulletin of the New York Academy of Medicine,* Vol 41, No 12 (December 1965).

Committee on the Costs of Medical Care. *Medical Care for the American People.* Chicago, University of Chicago Press, 1932. Republished under the title of *Medical Care for the American People* by the Department of Health, Education and Welfare, Public Health Service, Washington, DC, US Government Printing Office, 1970.

Comprehensive Community Health Services for New York City. New York, Commission on the Delivery of Personal Health Services, 1968.

*Comprehensive Health Planning, Selective Readings.* New York, Health

Insurance Institute, June 1969.

*Group Practice: Problems and Perspectives.* New York, New York Academy of Medicine, November 1968.

*Health Care in America.* Hearings before the US Senate Subcommittee on Executive Reorganization of the Committee on Government Operations. Washington, DC, US Government Printing Office, 1969.

Medical industrial complex. Health-Pac *Bulletin.* New York, Health Policy Advisory Center, November 1969.

*Medicare and Medicaid.* Hearings before the Committee on Finance, US Senate, 91st Congress, 2nd session, Parts I and II. Washington, DC, US Government Printing Office, 1970.

*Medicare and Medicaid: Problems, Issues, and Alternatives.* Report of the Staff to the Committee on Finance, US Senate. Washington, DC, US Government Printing Office, 1970.

National Commission on Community Health Services. *Health Is a Community Affair.* Cambridge, Mass., Harvard University Press, 1966.

Neighborhood health centers. *Medical Care,* Vol 8, No 2 (March-April 1970), entire issue.

Reed, L.S.: "Private health insurance, 1968, enrollment, coverage and financial experience. *Social Security Bulletin,* Vol 33, No 12 (December 1969), 19-25.

*Report of the National Advisory Commission on Health Manpower.* 2 Vols. Washington, DC, US Government Printing Office, November 1967.

Rice, D.P., Cooper, B.S.: National health expenditures, 1929-68. *Social Security Bulletin,* Vol 34, No 1 (January 1970), 3-20.

Somers, H.M., Somers, A.R.: *Medicare and the Hospitals.* Washington, DC, Brookings Institution, 1967.

Stevens, R.: *American Medicine and the Public Interest.* New Haven, Yale University Press, 1971.

US Department of Health, Education and Welfare. *Annual Reports.* Washington, DC: US Government Printing Office.

. *Financing Mental Health Care under Medicare and Medicaid.* Washington, DC, Social Security Administration, Research Report No 37, 1971.

. *Human Investment Programs: Delivery of Health Services to the Poor.* Washington, DC, US Government Printing Office, December 1967.

. *Report of the Task Force on Medicaid and Related Programs.* Washington, DC, US Government Printing Office, 1970.

. *Report on Licensure and Related Health Personnel Credentialing.* Washington, DC, Office of Assistant Secretary for Health and Scientific Affairs, Department of Health, Education and Welfare, June, 1971.

. *Task Force on Prescription Drugs, Final Report.* Washington, DC, US Government Printing Office, 1969.

Weinerman, E.R.: Research into the organization of medical practice. *Milbank Memorial Fund Quarterly,* Vol 44, No 4 (October 1966), Part 2, pp 104-145.

# PART 2

# THE OPTIONS AVAILABLE

# 3

# The Role of
# Government
# in the Health Services

## A Warning On Values

Because attitudes and values inevitably influence not merely an individual's decisions on policy but also his conception of the nature of the problem itself (i.e., his formal analysis) the reader should bear in mind certain of my preconceptions. The most relevant of these to the present discussion are:

First, I regard "government" as one of several possible institutions for achieving given ends. It is as "natural" in contemporary society as any other institution, whether it be the formally uncoordinated actions of individual consumers or producers (the institution of "private enterprise"), or an organized profession, or any other voluntary grouping of individuals to achieve ends for themselves or for others. From this perspective, therefore, the concept of government "intervention" or "interference" has no meaning, nor is "government" thought of as an agency for doing certain things that is utilized only as a "last resort." There are some things that are done better, and some worse, when the largest and most comprehensive unit of organization is involved. Utilizing government to achieve certain ends may entail some undesirable consequences as byproducts—just as the use of other institutions may do.

The question to be answered, therefore, is in what areas and aspects of the provision of health services (broadly interpreted) should the largest organizational unit of consumers participate and what should be the nature of its responsibilities? No final answer is offered here

Presented before the Committee on Social Policy for Health Care of the Committee on Special Studies of The New York Academy of Medicine, October 23, 1964, and published in the Bulletin of the New York Academy of Medicine, Vol XLI, No 7, July 1965. Reprinted by permission of the New York Academy of Medicine. Because this was written before the passage of the Social Security Amendments of 1965 there are no references to Medicare and Medicaid.

(although many of my own predilections will inevitably appear). Rather, the effort has been to lay out the issues and possible ways of grappling with them.

Second, I regard assurance of access to health services at the level that the nation is technically and economically able to provide for all its members an important goal of a democratic society. The importance attached to this objective stems from (1) the obvious significance of good health to the well-being and happiness of each individual, and (2) the bad economic and social consequences to society of the persistence of ill health among its members.

It is important to note that the formulation of this objective does not necessarily imply that health as a human need is necessarily more or less important than other kinds of needs (e.g., for income, education, decent housing, or legal service). The task before a group concerned with social policy for health is to spell out the institutional arrangements that would ensure access to the desired type and level of services and to indicate the demand that this provision would be likely to make on the national resources. It is for the community as a whole, and not for any professional group alone, to determine, in the light of the gains to be secured and economic costs involved, whether health has as high or a higher priority than certain other basic needs. At the same time it would seem highly appropriate for medical experts to give guidance to the community as to *priorities within the health field.*

Nor does the belief that access to appropriate health services should be available to all members of the community imply a commitment to any specific mechanism or set of arrangements for achieving the desired result. In particular, the formulation of the objective of access to the desired type and level of health services does not *necessarily* imply that health services should be provided as a free public service, like education. Such might be the conclusion but one could conceive of a society in which all incomes were sufficiently high to permit individuals to purchase needed services (individually or through insurance) from profit-making providers. And more realistically it is significant that different countries have adopted different approaches to the problem of ensuring adequate health care for their peoples, just as they have in meeting the problem of income maintenance, where we find a variety of mechanisms and programs both public and private rather than a single governmentally operated minimum income guarantee.

Third, I believe that the needed services must be made available to consumers under conditions that are "acceptable." Acceptability in my book has two aspects: the conditions under which it is available must not be offensive to individual dignity and self-respect and, insofar as technically possible, the consumer should be able to exercise choices as to the professionals serving him.

Consideration of both aspects involves judgments as to other people's values. On the first, I believe it has to be accepted that the vast majority of people in the United States dislike being the recipients of what they conceive to be charity, whether it be offered by an individual (as when a physician adjusts his fees to what he believes to be the income level of his patient) or by a philanthropic organization or by a government (as when any specific service is available only to persons who fall below some more or less explicitly defined measure of need). The strength of this feeling is most clearly evident in the widespread popularity of social insurance, here and in almost all major countries, for this is a mechanism for permitting the insured individual to claim benefits as a right and to feel that he has contributed toward their cost to the extent his means permit. The use of the word "claim" throws some light on what underlies this antipathy to charity, public or private. For it means that the individual who is a *claimant* is to a significant degree freed from dependence on the discretion of others (whether individuals or administrators of a program). He is no longer an "applicant." Thus the dislike of acceptance of charity is one aspect of the desire for freedom.

The desirable degree of freedom to choose the professional who will render service is more difficult to describe in general terms. Presumably it relates only to physicians, surgeons, dentists, and others rendering intimate personal service. For it should be noted that in vast areas of medical care freedom to select the individual practitioner does not even come into question. In hospitals patients cannot select their nurses (even with private-duty nurses it is a limited freedom). Nor do they select the intern or resident, and certainly not the renderers of auxiliary services (anesthesia, x-rays and many other treatments.) In outpatient and emergency facilities there is equally no free choice of doctor, and yet the use of these sources of medical care appears to be becoming more widespread and popular. And with the growth of "team" medicine it would seem that the freedom of the patient to select his individual professionals will be even more restricted, and that the values of his attempting to do so will be even more questionable.

Even in regard to the individual general practitioner, the surgeon, and the dentist, freedom of choice is severely circumscribed by the geographical availability of these professionals and by the incomes of those who seek care in relation to what they believe to be the charges of the professional.

There is perhaps no more useful service that a group of medical leaders could render toward a more rational consideration of the issues involved in the provision of health services than to clarify the meaning of the concept "freedom of choice of physician."

Fourth, as a professional person I have strong feelings about the importance of exclusive professional control of strictly professional matters. Differences of opinion on this topic seem to stem largely from different definitions of what is a "professional matter," and my own concept is undoubtedly narrower than that of the American Medical Association. Obviously it includes definition and evaluation of competence and quality of performance of professionals when only the profession can and should be the judge. I do not think it extends to arrangements for the organization and financing of health services. A profession would certainly be expected to evaluate different arrangements (actual or proposed) from the point of view of whether or not they are conducive to the rendering of high-quality service and to take a position accordingly. But I believe that no profession can set itself up as the arbiter of policy. In a democracy it is the community as a whole that in the last resort must determine policy—even if this means sacrificing maximum professional performance to some other objective.

Finally, it is probably hardly necessary to remind the reader that I am not a *medical* professional—what follows is written from the point of view of a consumer of health services who happens also to be a professional economist.

## The Extent of Government Involvement in the United States Prior to 1965

Even in the United States, where the role of government is probably less prominent than in almost all other countries of a comparable level of social and economic development, governments—federal, state, and local—are nevertheless heavily involved in the complex of arrangements for health care.

First, government already provides a sizable proportion of the total funds devoted to health care in the United States. Public expenditures accounted for 25.2% of all such expenditures, public, private consumers, and philanthropy, which amounted to approximately $32.9 billions in 1962-63. For personal health care alone (excluding such items as research, construction, etc.) the public share was 21.3% of a total of $28.6 billions. And, with the exception of the war and immediate postwar years, these proportions have sharply increased over the last 30 years. (The corresponding percentages in 1928-29 were 14.1 and 9.5.[1])

42

There has also been a shift in the respective roles of the federal government and the states. The former has been steadily increasing in importance. Of all *public* expenditures for health and medical care in 1934-35 the federal government contributed only 20.1%; the state and local share was 79.9%. By 1962-63 the federal share exactly equaled that of the states and localities.

The part played by government differs considerably in the different branches or areas of health care. As indicated above, governmental programs meet only a little over 20% of the expenditures for personal health care (hospitals and medical institutional care, physicians, and other professional services and drugs). The major programs for direct care are those provided and operated by the federal government for the armed forces and veterans, the special disease hospitals (mainly mental but some tuberculosis) financed and operated usually by the states and medical care programs for public assistance or other needy groups administered by states and/or localities but for which the federal government provides somewhat more than half the funds. Expenditures on other publicly financed programs, such as the program of health care of dependents of those in the armed forces and the health insurance program for federal employees (financed in part by the federal government but operated by private profit and nonprofit insurance agencies), maternal- and child-health services, medical care under workmen's compensation and vocational rehabilitation legislation, all have increased over the same period.

On the other hand, government provides almost two thirds of the funds devoted to medical and health-related research. Of an estimated total national expenditure for this purpose of $1.55 billions in 1962-63 government contributed no less than $1.018 billions (federal, $973 millions; state and local, $45 millions). Private expenditures accounted for only $532 millions (of which industry contributed $390 millions and philanthropy $142 millions).[1a]

In the construction of medical facilities the public share is less than that of the private sector ($632.5 millions as against an estimated $850 millions from private sources, including philanthropy).

Expenditures alone fail to give a full picture of the degree of governmental involvement in the provision of health care. For in general, government as a spender is unlikely to behave as an individual consumer who can exert little direct influence on the price charged, the quality of the care or the organizational arrangements for its provision (see below). Although there still appear to be some local public assistance authorities who foot the bill for medical care provided their clients without any concern at all for these matters, most governments in buying or subsidizing services lay down certain standards or requirements intended directly to affect prices of services, or quality or (less frequently) organization. And there may be considerable difference, too, in the total impact of any given volume of expenditures according to whether government acts through other agencies (philanthropic or profit-making) or whether it directly operates medical-care programs.

## The Problems as Viewed by Consumers
## (Including Would-Be Consumers)

From the viewpoint of the consumer the current arrangements for the provision of health services have many shortcomings.

### *Financial Restrictions on Access to Needed Health Services*
Although the health services have become more scientifically based and science has made possible more effective care, this progress has resulted in raising the costs of care to the individual or family. At the same time the population's expectations of the health service have increased. They believe that high levels of health are possible and their demand for health services has expanded correspondingly.

But the better service that is demanded (and in many cases supplied) costs money and, as incomes in general have not risen as fast as the costs of health care, the proportion of disposable personal income (income received by individuals less direct taxes paid by them) devoted to private consumer health expenditures has steadily increased. In 1948 these expenditures amounted to 4% of disposable personal income; by 1962 the percentage had risen to 5.7. In constant (1962) prices private consumers increased their per capita expenditures on medical care from $86.40 in 1948 to $119.44 in this same period.[2]

The rising costs and high level of care demanded have given rise to two acute problems: (1) because of their low levels of income, some segments of the population are unable to purchase needed care from their own resources at any time; and (2) because of the unequal incidence of illness and disability and the very high costs of some types of care, some individuals or families are either unable to meet the costs of some types of care, or do so only by exhausting their savings and/or contracting heavy debts.

*The role of the private sector.* The private sector of the economy has reacted to this situation in various ways:

(1) Adjustment of charges by the purveyor of service. Some

suppliers of medical services (notably the medical professions in the narrower sense) have adjusted their charges to what they know or believe to be the economic resources of their patients. But to the consumer this response has serious shortcomings:

• Although the medical profession does not seem aware of this, most patients find this form of private charity highly offensive and either do not seek care when they should, or avoid suppliers or forms of care believed to be "expensive," or accept the charity with resentment (which is hardly conducive to good doctor-patient relationships).

• To many members of the medical profession this introduction of financial bargaining into the patient relationship is distasteful. Furthermore, the inability of a patient to meet even the medically "reasonable" costs of various forms of treatment may deter a physician from prescribing what, as a medical man, he knows would be desirable. It is significant that in systems where the financing of medical care is no longer a matter for negotiation between individual doctor and individual patient, the favorable comment most frequently made by the participating physicians is that it is then possible to prescribe the medically indicated treatment without having to consider the patient's ability to pay for it.

Furthermore, there is a limit to the extent to which the physician can supply service to some patients at zero or below-market price, and the necessity to recoup himself by above-market charges to wealthier patients may meet resistance from them (even if he does not practice in a low-income neighborhood where rich patients are rare).

• Adjustment of charges by providers of service applies to part only of the consumers' medical care dollar (36.5% if dentists are also included). Adjustment of charges by the provider of service (or supplies) scarcely occurs in the sale of drugs, which accounts for 18.9% of consumer medical expenditure. And in hospital service, which commands 27.8% of the consumers' dollar, this type of adjustment appears to have become increasingly rare as hospital insurance has grown and as hospitals have exploited the possibilities of accepting needy patients via the public welfare system and charging at least part of the costs to some public agency.

(2) Development of private prepayment or insurance. A second type of adjustment in the private sector has taken the form of voluntary organization (initiated by consumers or, in the United States, more usually by producers) to develop systems of prepayment, most generally through the insurance mechanism. This approach has seen a dramatic expansion in the United States in the last thirty years. Insurance plans (Blue Cross and Blue Shield, commercial insurance, and

45

the independent plans providing specified health services on a group prepayment, risk-spreading basis) met 29.6% of the total personal health expenditure in 1962 (as against only 11.2% in 1948). The proportion varied greatly in the different branches of health care. Insurance payments in 1962 met 65.6% of hospital expenditures and only 33.6% of costs of physicians' services.[3]

From the consumers' standpoint, however, insurance, profit or non-profit, has certain disadvantages.

Voluntary insurance cannot be the answer for those consumers whose incomes are too low in any case to furnish the minimum requirements of decent living in the mid-20th century.

Thus, although three fourths of the population in the United States have some form of health-insurance coverage, it is significant that insurance has failed to make a serious impact on certain low-income groups such as migrants, low-income farmers, and the aged,[4] even though the low-income groups typically spend an above-average proportion of their incomes on medical care. In 1960-61, all urban families spent 6.6% of their incomes on medical care. Families with annual money incomes of under $2000 spent 8.2%, those with incomes of $2000 to $2999 spent 7.3%, and those with $4000 and more spent 6.4%.[5]

Furthermore, much of the great expansion of coverage in recent years has occurred in connection with the contract of employment. Those who are effectively out of the labor market are unlikely to be covered by this mechanism.

Efforts have been made by nonprofit concerns to expand the availability of insurance by setting community rates, averaging the costs of a high-risk group (e.g., the aged) over the entire group, and the like. But to do so necessitates raising premiums for the covered group and exposes segments of that group to the competitive appeal of commercial insurance companies which, by experience rating and selectivity of groups accepted, can offer more favorable terms to "good" risks. Thus it is not surprising that in recent years the commercial insurance companies have taken over a large share of the total of voluntary health insurance,[6] or that some of the nonprofit systems, e.g., Blue Cross in the city of New York, are departing from community rating.

The insurance industry in recent years has been making herculean efforts to meet the problem for one low-income group—the aged. Yet success has been limited, and some of the 65-plus plans are experiencing financial problems.

Even when the purchase of insurance is within the means of a consumer and he can find a plan to accept him, reliance on voluntary insurance is still an inadequate answer. For unless the scope of services provided for is wide, and unless the benefits assured take the form of service benefits, the consumer may still find himself carrying costs he regards as onerous.

Insurance is today still largely concentrated on the costs of acute care in hospitals and on surgical procedures; thus sizeable costs are not covered. The typical commercial insurance policy operates on the indemnity system and as, in general, the reimbursable sums are modest in relation to normal professional charges, the consumer may have a sizeable differential to meet, even if, despite consumer suspicions to the contrary, the provider of medical services does not deliberately increase his charges when he knows that the patient carries insurance.

Even under the most widespread nonprofit service plans, the Blue Cross and Blue Shield, the consumer is not completely covered. There are limits on the per diem reimbursement for room accommodation, and the shortage of semiprivate rooms in many hospitals means that the patient must meet the excess costs of single occupancy. (Here again consumers suspect that the providers of service on occasion have taken advantage of the availability of some insurance to make the patient buy a higher quality—and price—accommodation than he would wish.) Only very low-income receivers covered by Blue Shield plans are protected against additional charges by physicians over and above the amount reimbursed by the plan.

More recent efforts by private enterprise to meet the problem of "catastrophic" or unduly heavy medical expenses have undoubtedly been a real boon to the middle- and upper-income groups—until now. But it seems likely that an inherent feature of major medical insurance plans will, in the not-so-long run, limit and perhaps even reverse their rapid growth. This is the upward pressure on costs exerted by a system that exercises no control on the prices charged, and services prescribed, by suppliers of services from whom the brake of concern about the financial burden on their patients has been largely removed. The frequency with which major medical plans are finding it necessary to limit benefits or, more usually, to raise premiums, may well make this form of insurance financially unavailable to the income groups that need it most.

Finally, to the consumer, solution of the problem of financing medical care through the voluntary insurance mechanism carries with it certain costs. In 1962 the operating costs of all plans (meaning thereby the percentage that was retained for acquisition and other administrative expenses, premium taxes, additions to reserves and profits)

47

amounted to 14% of all payments for health insurance. The costs varied greatly for the different types of carrier.[7]

|  | Percent |
|---|---|
| Blue Cross-Blue Shield total | 7.2 |
| Blue Cross | 5.7 |
| Blue Shield | 11.0 |
| Insurance companies total | 20.0 |
| Group Insurance | 9.4 |
| Individual | 42.7 |
| Other plans | 9.2 |

*The role of government.* Far and away the most common type of governmental involvement (other than in the area of general "public health services" and of licensing, which will be dealt with below) is in regard to the financial inability of some groups to purchase needed care. Indeed, the history of most developed countries suggests that this problem has almost everywhere been the major stimulus to governmental involvement, and that public action in regard to the adequacy of facilities and personnel, the quality of care and the organizational arrangements for the provision of health services, and the economical use of resources has occurred primarily as a result of public involvement in the financing of personal health services.

In the latter area, governmental action has taken many forms:

(1) Meeting the costs of care for persons satisfying a needs test. This is the earliest type of public action to deal with the financial barriers to receipt of needed health services, and it is still the most widespread, although its actual importance in a country's total arrangements for the provision of medical care varies with the coverage of other governmental programs. In countries where medical care is freely available to all (e.g., in the Soviet Union and Great Britain) it plays no role. But even countries with extensive social insurance systems have found it necessary to provide, through public action, for the medical needs of the needy noninsured. In the United States this necessity accounted for approximately one seventh of all government expenditures for health and medical services in 1970.

Typically, needs-test medical care is administered by the public assistance authorities, who have adopted a variety of methods. In some cases the care is directly provided by the government itself, through a salaried physician or a governmentally owned and operated hospital. Sometimes it is purchased from organized suppliers (a contract may be made with a group of physicians, or hospital insurance may be

48

purchased through Blue Cross, for example). Sometimes the authority will merely pay the bills for services rendered to its clients, either meeting full cost or a fraction thereof, and this may be done either by direct payment to the supplier (the so-called vendor payment in public assistance programs in the United States) or (less frequently) by including an item for medical care in the budgets of public assistance recipients, who are then supposed to pay their own medical bills.

As a method of meeting the financial problems of individuals, means-test medical care has both advantages and disadvantages. As compared with all other methods (other than the universal public-service programs) it has the advantage of being, *in principle,* all-inclusive. It also meets the objections of those who ask why free medical care should be available to people who can easily afford to pay for it from their own resources.

But the all-inclusive potential is in practice limited by the fact that, except in Great Britain and New Zealand, which in any case have comprehensive health programs, public assistance is a locally administered program, and even in the United States it is a state rather than a joint responsibility in only about a dozen states and, in five of these, state responsibility does not extend to general assistance. The standards of eligibility and the nature and extent of care provided reflect local attitudes toward "the poor" as such, but even more the widely varying economic status of the local communities (and even states).

Thus there is great variation in both recipient rates and extent of care available under such systems,[8] and the problem is intensified because it is primarily the poorest and most depressed areas, where fiscal resources are least, which are likely to have the largest proportion of needy people.

Larger units of government have often been invoked to deal with the problem of unequal fiscal resources through the system of grants-in-aid (cf. the public assistance grants in the United States or the Kerr-Mills grant program). But because it has generally been thought necessary to require the recipient unit of government to carry some fraction of the costs as one method of ensuring responsible administration, the grant-in-aid still fails to overcome the financial problem faced by the poorest communities. And no grant-in-aid system has been able to overcome the obstacle to provision of adequate services that stems from local attitudes and values. Efforts to do so by requiring as a condition of receipt of a grant the provision of some minimum specified services (as under the Kerr-Mills law) does not achieve the desired result if a state simply decides that, on such conditions, it does not wish to accept the grant offer.

An even more serious disadvantage of means-test medical care is the fact that most people appear to find it psychologically offensive. It is significant that although some such program has been in effect since early times in most European and English-speaking countries, public pressure has led to the development of a wide variety of other arrangements (to be discussed below) to enable people to secure medical care without having to utilize "means-test medicine." In the United States efforts have recently been made, through the Kerr-Mills legislation, to create a "glorified" means-test medical-care program for the aged, but the evidence suggests that this is no more acceptable to those who found the means-test approach offensive, and that many who could benefit from it prefer not to do so. We do not know whether the same dislike of the program would prevail if (1) the test were administered by some authority other than the one administering public assistance, and (2) if eligibility were liberalized so as to eliminate the relatives' responsibility principle and to raise the income limit, which is today only slightly above the public assistance standard in most cases. But it should be noted that the more liberal the income test, the more such a program would approach a free public medical service.

A third disadvantage of means-test medical care is its impact on the nature and quality of the care available. When something is given as a concession the recipient typically has few rights, including the right to complain. Involvement with questions of quality and appropriateness of care is relatively rare on the part of the public assistance authorities. Given the prevailing attitude toward "the poor" a system of medical care thought of as "for the poor" is unlikely to be held to the same standards as apply to care paid for by the recipient, or available to the entire population as a public service (such as education). It is significant that many observers of the British Health Service attribute the many improvements, from the patient's point of view, that have been effected since 1948, to the fact that for the first time the middle classes are the users of public medical care and are demanding the kind of standards and quality to which they have been accustomed. It is no longer a service "for the poor only."

(2) Granting subsidies to institutions organized by private in- dividuals to lighten or remove the financial burden for themselves or others. Governments have utilized the subsidy principle in various ways:

• Subsidies to consumer-organized prepayment systems. In a number of European countries during the 19th century, groups of workers, trade unions, or citizens of a given community organized mutual benefit or sickness funds to pay for the medical care of their members. An early form of public action was the encouragement of such activity by the granting of subsidies to permit these organizations to pay for a wider range of service, or to enroll less affluent members, or to equalize financial burdens as between rich and poor or healthy and unhealthy communities. Despite governmental encouragement and growing subsidies, these organizations failed to attain acceptable coverage or to meet the costs of a full range of health services, and one country after another has replaced the subsidized voluntary system by compulsory health insurance as the only way to ensure appropriate coverage and in view of the fact that even the subsidy system involved a high degree of governmental control. For as public financial participation increased it was accompanied by increasingly specific standards which extended beyond safeguards for accountability to the minimum types of services to be insured against, or the membership eligibility conditions.

• Subsidies toward the purchase of private insurance (nonprofit or commercial). Proposals for this type of government action have been under discussion in the United States in recent years as an alternative to a public compulsory hospitalization insurance program for the aged. In fact, relatively few countries or states appear to have adopted this approach.

Australia is a notable exception.[9] People insure with a private insurance organization for specified benefits. For medical care, in addition to their insurance benefit they receive a Commonwealth Benefit from the federal government on the basis of a fee-for-service schedule. For hospitalization, the patient receives, in addition to his private insurance benefit, two subsidies from the government: a daily payment (8/−) paid to every patient insured or not, plus a second daily payment of 12/− if he is insured.

Despite the stimulus given to insurance and extensive advertising, the scheme after 13 years had enrolled only about 70% of the population. And for those covered not all costs are met. Medical men are free to charge whatever they wish, and the total refund (insurance plus the government benefit) has represented between 63 and 64% of medical fees paid in recent years. For hospital care the freedom of the insured person to select the amount of coverage he will purchase makes generalization more difficult, but it is believed that even with the substantial public subsidy, many insured individuals are not fully protected.

It is important to note, too, that this program is buttressed by other public medical programs. A separate pharmaceutical benefits system, universally available, provides for reimbursement of the cost of drugs in excess of 5/— per prescription. There is also a program of special daily subsidies for nursing and convalescent homes, whose long-stay inmates typically have exhausted their insurance benefits. And there is a pensioner medical service which provides free medical care to pensioners and their dependents under a special means test, the physicians being reimbursed by the government.

● Subsidies to philanthropy. In most countries organized philanthropy has played a more or less important role in the provision of health services. The church in earlier days in Europe and, more recently, private sectarian and nonsectarian charitable groups have built and operated hospitals, financed health services such as visiting nurse services, and financed treatment and research for specific types of illness (polio, mental retardation, cancer, etc.). In some countries, such as the United States, government has encouraged their development by granting subsidies in the form of tax concessions, both to the private individual who contributes to them and to the organized institution or agency that operates as a nonprofit corporation.

In fact, despite this substantial encouragement, the role of philanthropy appears to be diminishing (except perhaps in hospital construction). Furthermore, as a method of overcoming the general problem of the financial barrier to access to medical health services, philanthropy has several disadvantages. It tends to be spotty in coverage, concentrating on specific illnesses that have a dramatic public appeal but not very broad incidence. Where, as in the case of the private general hospital, no such "disease selectivity" prevails in principle, it may be replaced by other types of selectivity. In a publicly operated service the potential clients are defined by law, the public agency must accept all who fulfill the legal eligibility conditions, even if it means lowering standards of care because of limited resources, and it is held responsible when eligible persons are not served. But the subsidized private agency is not so constrained. It can pick and choose among those who wish to use its services and it may reject some either because of a desire to maintain high standards in the face of limited income or because the patients may be regarded as inappropriate subjects for research or teaching.

The subsidized private agency thus tends to encourage the development of two systems of care, and the higher the quality of care rendered by the protected voluntary system, the more is this likely to be true. It is interesting to note that precisely the same situation prevails in social work, another service industry characterized by considerable reliance on private philanthropy, especially in the North and the East. Here we find a sharp division: high-standard voluntary agencies attracting the cream of the professionals interested in high-quality practice and research, serving a very limited clientele who are selected by reference to whether their diagnosed needs fit the agencies' own defined purposes and who are to an increasing degree middle class. On the other hand, we find the public welfare agencies swamped with heavy case loads, many of them among the most difficult and needy cases and, because of the necessity to ration service not by turning people away, but by giving limited or perfunctory service to each, unable to attract well-trained professionals.

• Subsidies to individual consumers. In the United States, government has been invoked to assist the individual in meeting his medical bills by granting income-tax deductions for medical expenditures. This approach has serious shortcomings. On the one hand, it gives no assistance at all to the person whose income and other claimable deductions place him below the taxable income level. Thus it fails to solve the problem for some groups for whom it is most acute (e.g., the aged, the poor, and large families). And on the other hand it gives most help to those who need it least, namely, the very rich. For the dollar value of a deduction in a progressive tax system is greatest to the man whose income is taxed at the highest marginal rate. A tax *credit* would avoid this disadvantage, but the first one would still remain. In the United States abolition of this concession would, it is estimated, increase federal revenues by $1.16 billions (based on 1963 incomes at 1965 tax rates). It is thus a sizeable subsidy. All but $200 million of this is claimed by persons with adjusted gross incomes in excess of $5000.

*Compulsory insurance.* Apart from public assistance, this is far and away the most common governmental method of attacking the financial obstacle to receipt of health services. Individuals and, almost universally in the case of wage-earners, their employers are required to pay ear-marked taxes (euphemistically and for historical reasons called contributions) in return for which they (and usually their families) are entitled to receive care free or on a subsidized basis. In many cases the government also contributes from general revenues to the health insurance fund.

Essentially the same approach is found in New Zealand where, although "social insurance contributions" are not found, income-receivers are required to pay an additional, ear-marked income tax in return for which they are entitled to certain types of health services. However here, as in Norway and Sweden, where a universal compulsory health insurance system prevails, the right to receive medical care on a free or subsidized basis is not conditional on having in fact paid the required contributions or taxes.

Within this general framework there is great variation among the different systems.

• Coverage of the programs. Among the insurance systems, properly so-called (excluding the Norwegian, Swedish, and New Zealand systems), none provides for universal coverage. The insurance concept implies that entitlement to benefits is established by the prior payment of the taxes for some specified period. Individuals who have no incomes to tax or who are not employed, or whose conditions of employment are likely to make the technical tax collection problem very difficult, are either excluded by intent or in fact (migrant workers and certain types of agricultural and domestic workers). Certain groups are sometimes covered by separate and somewhat differently financed plans (agricultural employees, farmers, and the self-employed), and sometimes provision is made for voluntary insurance. Family members are usually covered as dependents of the insured person. Coverage of European insurance systems ranges between 16.3% of the population (Greece) or 17% (Portugal) to 82.4% (West Germany), the most usual percentage being between 45 and 55.[10]

Sometimes there are income limits to coverage, those with wages or incomes above a certain limit being excluded.

• Range of health benefits provided. Although the tendency everywhere is for wider coverage, most systems limit in some degree the types or the duration of care. The British system (1911-1948) was essentially limited to general practitioner services. In some systems, especially if the country is provided with a free or otherwise financed hospital system, hospitalization may be excluded. Dental benefits are not always available, or they are restricted to certain population groups, such as children and expectant mothers. Pharmaceuticals, sometimes on a restricted basis, are usually included among the benefits. Prostheses may or may not be provided.

In some cases, as in Canada, social insurance has been applied only in regard to hospitalization, although the recent Royal Commission report recommends its extension to cover all medical services.[11]

• Utilization of the reimbursement or the service principle. Some systems reimburse the patient (or the supplier of the services) with some fraction of the costs incurred, or with full cost, based upon some legally specified tariff. This is the case, for example, in Sweden, Norway, New Zealand, Australia, and France. Others make the defined services freely available to the insured person and pay the suppliers directly (according to a variety of principles and methods to be referred to below), so that the patient has no financial dealings of any kind with the vendor. This was the policy in Great Britain from 1911 to 1948 under the health insurance system, and it prevails today in Italy and Germany (except for some drugs for family members). In some cases this system is modified by the imposition of a (usually nominal) charge for certain goods or services (drugs, dentures, eyeglasses, etc.).

As a technique for removing the financial barrier it is evident that, to the consumer, the service approach is the more effective. For unless the vendors agree not to charge more than the charges specified in the tariff, the consumer still has to meet the difference between what is reimbursed and what the professional supplier charges, and this may be considerable.[12] And unless reimbursement is at the 100% rate he will always have to bear some of the cost. This greatly limits the effectiveness of the program to the low-income receiver and necessitates the utilization of some additional machinery (usually on a means-test basis) if such people are to secure the care they need. The advantage claimed for partial reimbursement only is, of course, that it acts as a brake on irresponsible use of the service—to which it has been objected that it may equally deter individuals from seeking care until a condition becomes acute and thus works against early detection and possible prevention.

• Methods of supplying health care. Most health insurance systems involve a minimum of intervention in the existing organizational arrangements for providing medical care. The patient uses such doctors or hospitals or clinics as he chooses among those available in his community and willing to participate in the program, and the only difference is in the financial realm. The insurance system usually has little concern with quality of care except to provide safeguards against gross incompetence and provision of grievance machinery for dissatisfied patients, and none at all with the adequacy and distribution of personnel and facilities. On the other hand, there are likely to be efforts to control quality of care as it affects cost (see below). Essentially the position is that if an individual can secure medical attention the system will relieve him of some or all of the costs.

Some systems, however, provide the legally specified services directly, though these usually take the form of special institutions such as convalescent homes, sanatoria, and the like. But in Austria the insured person must seek care from doctors under contract in health establishments (dispensaries and hospitals) belonging to the several insurance institutions.

• Methods of remunerating professional suppliers. Because most compulsory insurance systems purchase care from professionals in private practice or from public or private hospitals and similar institutions, the financial arrangements have assumed great importance—unfortunately often to the exclusion or neglect of other aspects of governmental involvement in the provision of health services.

For professional services the insurance fund typically negotiates methods of payment with representatives of the medical profession (or with a group representing the doctors who are willing to participate in the program). A wide variety of payment systems is to be found, the more important of which will be discussed in Chapter 4.[13] With hospitals or clinics the financial arrangements may be negotiated either with the institutions as a group or individually (in the latter case usually within the limits of a scale set by the central authority).

In the case of both individual practitioners and institutions these negotiations have often given rise to sharp differences of opinion between the suppliers of service and the social insurance authority.[14] (Because the essential problems are the same, similar differences have arisen in the case of a national health service.)

● Methods of financing. Although all social insurance systems collect taxes or contributions from potential beneficiaries (and/or their employers) the extent to which these funds meet all costs of the system varies from country to country. Not infrequently the contributions are supplemented by funds from the general revenues. A few countries, however, provide for no public subsidy to the general scheme although the state may contribute funds to schemes for special groups (such as miners in Austria, or students in West Germany, the severely disabled and war survivors in France, etc.).

Care must be taken in generalizing about the extent of contributions from the general taxpayer to allow for the fact that in some countries important types of health services are directly provided by government outside the insurance system. Thus in Sweden, in addition to certain subsidies to the social insurance system itself, much medical care is furnished through the hospital system, for which the health insurance funds pay only a nominal sum, the remainder being financed by the owners and operators of the hospitals (90% of them being public authorities in Sweden).

● General limits to the social insurance approach. Some of the achievements and shortcomings of the compulsory insurance approach in regard to quality of care and use of resources will be dealt with in subsequent pages. But as a method of removing the financial barrier to receipt of health services it should be noted that social insurance has two serious disadvantages. First, unless it takes the form (as in New

Zealand, Norway, or Sweden) of a universally applicable requirement to "insure" or to pay taxes coupled with arrangements for blanketing-in (usually at the expense of the general taxpayer) groups not, in fact, paying the tax or contribution, it fails to provide universal coverage. Second, as a method of financing it is distinctly regressive. The worker's share is at best a proportionate tax with no deductions or exemptions, there is often a ceiling on taxable wages, and the employer's share is generally held to be in large measure shiftable via wages or prices. Whether or not this is a serious disadvantage depends on the progressive or nonprogressive character of other parts of the tax structure, and the presence or absence of some subsidy from general revenues to the health insurance system. In the United States, where all other social insurance programs are financed wholly from wage and/or payroll taxes, this might be a serious consideration although, even so, it could be argued that if the insurance approach is to be utilized social insurance has at least the advantage, as compared with private insurance, of assessing charges that are in some measure proportionate to income.

*Direct provision of some or all types of health services for some or all members of the community.* This kind of governmental responsibility, which involves employing professionals and owning and operating facilities, has been accepted in varying degrees:

● For some types of illness. Thus in the United States, as in many other countries, institutional care for those with mental illness, tuberculosis, or leprosy has typically been provided in public hospitals—perhaps because such people were regarded as constituting a danger to the community and public action was regarded as a form of police action or "public health" activity.

● For some types of services. Apart from environmental health services the most usual type of health service undertaken by government is hospitalization. Thus in Norway and Sweden hospital care is an almost free service universally available in publicly owned and operated hospitals.

● Comprehensive care for some groups. In the United States, government has sole responsibility for ensuring receipt of needed health services for members of the army, for veterans with service-connected disabilities and, to an increasing degree, especially for hospitalization, for veterans with nonservice-connected disabilities. This kind of publicly provided care is also available to members of Congress, presidents, and other important officials.

● Comprehensive care for the entire population. Outside the

Communist countries, Great Britain is the only major country to expand the role of government to embrace acceptance of full responsibility for ensuring free medical care (subject only to certain modest charges for dentures, eyeglasses and drugs) and needed health services to all members of the community, regardless of the payment of prior contributions or the passage of a test of need, or even of citizenship. The National Health Service (NHS) owns and operates practically all facilities and employs 95% of the professionals. Although a small number of institutions remain in private hands for the utilization of those who do not wish to avail themselves of the public facilities, and although general practitioners, specialists, and dentists are permitted to accept private patients, only about 5% of health care is in fact received "outside the service." This approach is, of course, the only certain and complete answer to the problem of the financial barrier to receipt of medical care. And it is an answer that does not involve either the passage of a needs test (a relatively few individuals who find the payment of the charges for drugs, etc., a hardship can secure reimbursement from the National Assistance Board on passage of the Board's test of need) or the organization of health services into two systems, one for "the poor" and one for the rich. It is equally obvious that the comprehensiveness and quality of care available depends on the extent to which government assures an adequate supply and distribution of personnel and facilities and on other factors affecting quality of care (see below). At the very least the national health service approach involves a rationing of available facilities and personnel by some principle other than ability to pay.

## Difficulties of Securing High Quality and Appropriate Care for Other than Financial Reasons

Despite the great advances in medical technology, there is a sizeable gap between the quality and level of health care many people receive and the care that is technically possible. A major complaint of consumers is indeed that even when financial considerations are not a major obstacle they are not always or everywhere able to secure high quality care. This is due to several factors:

*Inadequacies in the supply of personnel and facilities in general or in certain geographical areas.* There is considerable difference of opinion as to the adequacy of the total supply of medical personnel and facilities in the United States.[15] Although the number of physicians per 100,000 population has been declining (there was a slight increase after 1957) it is held that this has been largely offset by rising productivity, including both greater technical efficiency and a higher ratio of patients actually cared for per physician. However, the latter may merely indicate an adaptation to scarcity. Certainly to the consumer the shorter time spent with the doctor, the declining frequency of home visits, the necessity to staff some hospitals with doctors trained abroad (some of dubious competence), and the fact that physicians' incomes have increased more sharply than those of other professional groups—all these factors indicate scarcity relative to demand and a deficiency in the output of medical graduates. Whatever views may be held as to the adequacy of the total supply of personnel and facilities, there is no gainsaying the fact that some parts of the country are better supplied than others, and conversely.[16]

● The role of the private sector. The principles on which the private sector operates would suggest that the free market would ensure a supply commensurate with demand. Scarcity would lead to high prices for the scarce service or facility and this, in turn, would stimulate a transfer of resources to the items in short supply. In the health services this operates only to a limited degree, because:

○ The high cost of training for professional service, which limits access to professional schools, narrows the area of recruitment. The lower income groups are in no position to respond to the high market value of professional service and, in fact, are very poorly represented among practitioners.

○ Entry to the professions is controlled by organized professions which, for otherwise good and understandable reasons, are granted a legal monopoly. Although formally their authority relates only to the determination of professional competence it can, in effect, extend to the supply of training facilities (as when an influential medical association opposes the creation of additional medical schools). Effective control by a private organization of entry to a profession can operate well or badly to ensure an appropriate total supply, depending on whether the profession concerned places predominant emphasis on the individual economic interest of its members (which are of course served by scarcity) or on the well-being and needs of the community. (To the nonmedical observer there seems to be a sharp difference between, for example, the medical and the nursing professions in the United States in this respect.)

Private philanthropy has also played a role in the problem of supply and distribution of health services. Through scholarships and other training grants and by supplying funds for the construction of facilities (mainly hospitals) some contribution has been made to a better supply and, perhaps to a lesser degree, to distribution of personnel and facilities. But, as pointed out earlier, the role of philanthropy, in global terms, is not large.

Whatever the degree of success the private sector may have in ensuring an appropriate total supply of medical personnel and facilities, it has notably failed to ensure a geographically even distribution. In the case of physicians this reflects the freedom of the professional to locate in areas where he believes there is likely to be an effective demand for his services (i.e., one backed by an ability to pay) and, probably more importantly, in areas where there exist appropriate facilities (hospitals, laboratories, ancillary services, research centers) that will enable him to practice high quality medicine. The professional seeks, too, the stimulus of a group of colleagues. This largely explains the relative scarcity of physicians in rural low-income areas and their high concentration in the metropolitan areas.[17] It is noteworthy that in these preferences medical men are not different from those in other professional groups who are motivated by the same desire to do work of high professional quality; the same type of maldistribution—giving rise to the same kind of social concern—is found among social workers and university professors.

● The role of government. People have used their governments to overcome the problems of supply and distribution in various ways:

○ Supply of public funds to encourage training of personnel and construction of facilities. Even in countries such as the United States, where government is not actively involved in the provision of medical care (other than to its own employees and a few special groups), this kind of action is found. The Hill-Burton Hospital Construction Act, the Mental Health legislation, the recently passed Nursing Act, all involving either construction and/or training grants, are illustrations of this type of action—in this case by the offer of grants by the federal government to states and to nonprofit organizations. A similar quite comprehensive program was adopted in Canada in the National Health Grants Program of 1948.

In the United States this type of action has been especially noteworthy in regard to the production of knowledge and the training of research workers. The stimulus there has taken the form both of direct public operation (as in the various National Institutes of Health) and grants to public and nonprofit organizations for research and training.

In a national health service such as the British, all initiative in the supply area is of course in the hands of government. On the one hand this approach has the advantage of ensuring a comprehensive evaluation of both total and relative needs (e.g., for different types of professionals or facilities, as well as geographical differentials) because "the government" is held responsible for inadequacies. The National Health Service (NHS) in Britain, for example, has made noteworthy strides in grappling with the still serious shortage of nurses, although it has made less progress in regard to the shortage of dentists.

But sole public responsibility has also certain disadvantages, or social costs. Concentration of control of supply in the hands of a single authority means that a wrong decision can have serious consequences. Thus the decision of the British government to cut by 10% the entrants to medical schools, following the recommendations of the Willink Committee a few years ago, has proved to have been an unfortunate underestimate of total medical needs, and shortages are already developing.

To both the professions involved and to the government, centralization of responsibility for ensuring an adequate supply of personnel for the health services has the troublesome consequence of involving government in the determination of the terms and conditions of employment. For it is not merely a matter of attracting and retaining an appropriate total supply: the relative supplies of different kinds of professionals are also involved (general practitioners versus specialists, different types of specialists, etc.). The story of the negotiations of the British government with the various medical groups since 1948 indicates the complexity of these problems.[18] At the same time, it must be recognized that the problem of appropriate price relationships among various types of medical personnel has not always been satisfactorily solved when decisions are left to the private sector, and governmental decision-making has at least the advantage of bringing the issues into the open.

Finally, where the decision to allocate more or less of national resources to the health services is made centrally by government, the health services are necessarily evaluated in relation to other national needs. From the national standpoint this is, of course, desirable, but it may mean that at times the health services are accorded a lower priority than they might have secured if the decision to increase supply had been left to the private sector. The failure of the British for the first thirteen to fourteen years of the Health Service to construct any significant number of new hospitals is a case in point (the situation is now being remedied). And, in a country with powerful sectional or other organized pressure groups, governmental decisions as to the supply and, more particularly, the location of facilities may reflect political pressure rather than rationally determined need (e.g., the supply and location of veterans' hospitals in the United States).

○ Measures to control the geographical maldistribution of facilities and personnel. Governments have sometimes dealt with the problem of acute shortage of personnel and facilities, especially in isolated areas, by direct employment of professionals and provision of facilities in these areas. Thus, in Sweden, where for geographical reasons this problem is acute, there has long been a system of salaried district medical officers who both oversee health conditions in their areas, provide direct medical care and, on occasion, direct small hospitals. In the western provinces of Canada isolated communities have formed hospital districts to erect and maintain hospitals out of public funds. In Saskatchewan the inability of isolated rural areas to attract private physicians led to the development of the municipal doctor system whereby a doctor is hired from public funds to provide general practitioner service, a system that considerably expanded after 1939 until it was replaced by the comprehensive Medical Care Program in 1962. To a lesser extent this system has also been used in Alberta and Manitoba.

Another approach available under social insurance or national health services has been to offer special inducements to doctors to practice in otherwise unpopular areas. These may take the form of higher remuneration and other privileges. But they may also take the form of efforts to meet the professional's dislike of the other conditions affecting his work, by constructing, or encouraging the construction of, medical facilities, or by promoting further training and contact with research-oriented colleagues by special leave programs and additional payments for educational leave.

A third technique for correcting the maldistribution of physicians has been adopted for general practitioner service in Great Britain and is known as "negative control." A doctor who desires to practice under the NHS may not do so in an area that has been classified by a national Medical Practices Committee (seven of whose nine members are general practitioners) as "overdoctored" although he is free to practice anywhere he wishes as a private practitioner. The effectiveness of this technique depends of course on the coverage of the public program and the importance attached by professionals to the privilege of being associated with it.

Where health services are directly operated by a government that both owns the facilities and directly employs the professionals, maldistribution can be directly dealt with by decisions as to the location of facilities and the size and composition of their staff. It is generally agreed, for example, that since 1948, the NHS in Britain has

62

brought about a considerable improvement in the distribution of specialists who, if operating under the service, are employed on a salaried (sessional) basis in the public hospitals.

It is indeed difficult to see how the problem of maldistribution can be resolved without the direct involvement of government. The resources of the thinly populated or poorer areas must be supplemented if they are to offer the remuneration and, more importantly, the other conditions of employment that appeal to professionals. And it is doubtful whether reliance on economic inducements alone will correct the situation. Even in Sweden, where there is a very comprehensive public hospital system and a method of remunerating doctors that attempts to reflect geographical differences and types of responsibility, there is a heavy concentration of professionals in Stockholm. And in Norway, where the comprehensive insurance system pays doctors on a fee-for-service basis, the otherwise highly enthusiastic director general of health services has to admit that the system does not guarantee an equal distribution of doctors throughout the country, and that the problem is especially acute in regard to specialists.[19]

In Britain there has been little improvement in the geographical distribution of dentists, in contrast to that in the general practitioner and specialist services where some controls, as indicated above, have been applied.

*Other obstacles to securing appropriate high quality care.* Even where medical personnel and facilities abound and even where the consumer possesses an "adequate" income he cannot be sure that he is in fact obtaining appropriate and high quality medical care. Unlike the consumer of automobiles, food, clothing, etc., the purchaser of medical care offered on the open market is often a poor judge of good or bad quality and of the appropriateness of one type of treatment or care versus another, while the consequences of a mistaken choice may be infinitely more serious. This is, of course, because such judgments call for training and technical knowledge not possessed by the nonprofessional. The plight of the consumer is intensified by the development of specialization among the professionals and by the uncoordinated nature of current institutional arrangements for the supply of health services. Where dissatisfaction exists, the consumer is frustrated in many cases by the absence of any machinery for ventilating complaints and having power to remedy the situation.

● The role of the private sector. Some safeguards are, of course, provided in the private sector:

○ In any market where goods and services are supplied by private enterprise, control over quality and appropriateness is supposed to be assured by consumer preferences selecting among competing suppliers. In the provision of health services, however, this mechanism operates only to a limited degree. Even if the consumer has the knowledge to distinguish between "good" and "bad" care, his control is severely limited.

First, difficulties are faced by the individual in changing his source of supply. If a patient is dissatisfied with his physician, what other one does he choose? Unlike sellers in the commodity market, suppliers of medical care do not advertise their wares and their good points (and by implication the bad points of competitors). Medical etiquette even denies the consumer benefit of expert judgment of one professional by others—and also places psychological obstacles in the way of a change of physician.

Second, insofar as institutional services go, the consumer, at the time he needs such care, is scarcely in a position to exercise choice. In any case, here he faces the problem of joint supply. He uses those facilities that are available to the surgeon or physician who treats him. In many communities there is only one hospital or other facility.

Third, the final control exercised by the individual consumer lies in the possibility of bringing damage suits. These actions have increased markedly in recent years. But their usefulness as an instrument for assuring appropriate and high quality care is questionable. The cost of bringing action is likely to deter many dissatisfied individuals. The outcome is uncertain, in part due to the professional solidarity of the suppliers of services. The growth of insurance against such actions on the part of professionals may yield sizeable damages to the aggrieved patient, but the deterrent effect upon the incompetent physician of the fear of a suit is likely to be weakened. Finally, fear of such suits, as suggested below, may encourage overuse of certain medical resources.

It might have been expected that group action by consumers would have exercised control over appropriateness and quality. But this seems to have occurred only to a limited degree. Consumer information services, similar to those evaluating quality and price of other consumer items, do not exist except occasionally in regard to certain drugs. Organized purchasers of care and services, such as the nonprofit and commercial insurance companies, have in general refrained from involvement in the appropriateness and quality of service, although they are increasingly concerned about the quantity and cost of care.

The lack of involvement in appropriateness and quality on the part of the major organizations paying for care in the United States is probably not unrelated to the fact that they originated with suppliers of care or as a profit-making venture, and their management typically contains little or no consumer representation. Only in the consumer-organized or initiated programs, such as union-negotiated plans or some group-health plans, does the consumer have the power to evaluate and, possibly, to do something about, quality. Yet even in the union-negotiated plans, involvement with questions of quality and organization for the provision of health services has been limited.[20]

○ To a very considerable extent the private sector today relies on the medical profession to deal with problems of appropriateness and quality. The assumption is that the patient will select a general practitioner (who as a licensed physician presumably possesses some approved level of competence) who will normally refer the patient elsewhere for such services as he himself cannot provide. But this system has serious shortcomings.

First, the general practitioner may himself not be highly competent. He may indeed possess the minimum qualifications required for licensing at the time he was licensed. But with the rapid growth of medical knowledge the general practitioner of yesterday may not be qualified today. Those who have access to hospitals, especially teaching hospitals, are more likely to keep in touch with new developments, and certainly they have the advantage of available consultants. But this is not the case for the doctor in less well-equipped communities. In regard to the increasingly technical field of drugs, antibiotics, etc., the evidence suggests that to a large extent the physician is "educated" by representatives of the drug manufacturers supplemented by evaluations in the professional journals. The consumer can hardly feel that this is likely to lead to the most effective prescriptions,[21] nor has his confidence in professional evaluations been reinforced by recent revelations. In any case, the average practitioner's work load is such that the time he can devote to professional study must be severely limited. (This may be another indication of the scarcity of doctors.)

Second, not every individual or family uses a "family physician." This is due in part to financial considerations, but it also seems likely to reflect some loss of confidence in the professional competence of the average general practitioner. To an increasing degree patients appear to make some of their own diagnoses and select their own specialists.

The medical profession is also entrusted by society with the policing of performance by its own members. There seems to be general agreement that where a large number of medical professionals function within the confines of a given institution this kind of "peer control" can be highly effective, although there are instances to the contrary.

But this kind of control can hardly operate in sparsely-doctored areas and, in general, its effectiveness among solo-practicing general practitioners is probably limited.

There is, moreover, considerable evidence that the "ethics" or, at least, the "etiquette" of the profession serves to limit the extent to which it does indeed police itself. The extent of abuse by medical men in certain Workmen's Compensation systems, unchecked by the profession itself, is well known. The reluctance of doctors to testify against colleagues is understandable, but hardly conducive to enforcement of professional standards.

● The role of government. Public action to ensure high quality and appropriateness has taken several forms:

○ Control of the quality of certain types of service or supplies. Reference has already been made to the fact that where the welfare of the individual will be threatened by incompetent practice, governments typically require the practitioner to obtain a license to practice, which is granted on the basis of a test of competence. The professionals applying the test may be directly employed by government or, more usually, responsibility is delegated to a recognized professional organization.

To a growing extent the same concern appears to be extending to institutions, although the control is not so rigid or so widespread.[22] Compliance with the standards of privately organized professional accrediting bodies may not be legally required as a condition of continued operation, but if government plays a large role in the organization or financing of health services it may be enforced de facto. Participation in, e.g., a health insurance system may be limited to accredited hospitals or nursing homes. Public assistance authorities may reimburse the costs of medical care provided their clients only if supplied by an accredited institution.

Another type of control of quality is represented in this country by the Food, Drug and Cosmetic Acts, and similar arrangements exist elsewhere.

○ Measures affecting the physician's relationship to his patients. Two elements entering into the concept of "quality of care" have always been of great concern to the medical profession when contemplating compulsory health insurance systems or national health services. They are the freedom of the patient to choose his doctor and the freedom of the doctor to treat his patient without third-party intervention.

In the democracies, almost all public programs that have wide coverage permit the patient to select his own general practitioner and to change if dissatisfied. This is obvious in such schemes as the Australian system of subsidizing private insurance, which interferes not at all with the traditional methods of operation of medical men and hospitals. But it occurs, too, in almost all compulsory insurance systems. Even though the patient may be required to use a doctor who has agreed to participate in the program, the fact that in most countries there is extensive participation gives the patient a wide measure of choice, probably far wider than would be available to those of low or modest income in the absence of compulsory insurance. In some countries using the reimbursement system, the patient is permitted to use professionals or institutions other than those entering into agreements with the government, but he is reimbursed only up to, or occasionally below, the legal tariff. In universal coverage systems or a national health service free choice is even more certainly ensured. Although doctors are free not to participate in the program, indirect pressure from patients ensures that most of them do.

The major areas in which government's concern with costs has involved any interference with the doctor-patient relationship are the use of drugs and of hospitals. All the evidence suggests that in general public authorities are almost excessively careful not to interfere in the direct patient-doctor relationship and that frequently they confine themselves to admonition, to advisory circulars, and to public reports. Even where more direct controls are applied, the public administrators have attempted to operate through professional organizations or channels. Thus in Great Britain, when administrative records indicate that certain doctors are grossly out of line in regard to the volume of prescriptions, disciplinary action is taken by the local executive councils, which consists primarily of medical men. Similarly, suspected overuse of hospitals may be met by a requirement for the formation of a professionally staffed utilization committee in each hospital.

The desire to control unnecessary prescribing, or the use of expensive proprietary drugs in place of cheaper and equally efficient prescriptions sometimes leads to the policy of publishing lists of drugs that can be freely prescribed, and listing others for which permission must be secured from some designated medically staffed committee. Some doctors regard this as an undue interference in their professional functioning.[23] Even where the pressure to control costs or the need to correct abuse or gross malpractice causes a public authority (e.g., the social insurance agency or the administrator of a national health service) to question the treatment given to an individual patient, the officials conducting the investigation are always medical men. In general, however, the evidence suggests that this type of supervision of an individual practitioner's judgment occurs primarily in relation to the certification of inability to work in the case of workers claiming disability insurance cash benefits, rather than in regard to the program concerned with provisions of health services per se.

○ The impact of specific financial arrangements on quality. Financial considerations and specific financial arrangements with suppliers of care can and sometimes have exerted an adverse effect on quality.

Unwillingness of the community to provide through the tax system total sums adequate to provide high quality health services may lower quality in various ways. Failure to invest sufficient public funds to train and equip an adequate supply of professional personnel may lead to unduly long patient lists and perfunctory service. Failure to devote adequate resources to public hospitals (as happened in Great Britain until recently) means long waiting lists and crowded conditions—as it does in the City of New York.

Arrangements for the remuneration of practitioners can and have also affected quality. Failure to set levels of remuneration that in general compare favorably with those for professions or employments calling for comparable skills and training may cause the public service to face difficulty in attracting and retaining an appropriate supply of medical personnel. Differential levels of remuneration that place the specialist (as in Great Britain) at an advantage as compared with the general practitioner may drain personnel away from an essential service, although if (as also in Great Britain) government controls specialist appointment to hospitals, the grosser effects can be avoided. Where both public and private systems prevail, low levels of remuneration and unsatisfactory working conditions in public hospitals may result in a lowered quality of public hospital staffs.

Where fee-for-service systems operate, the relative payments for different medical acts or procedures may have an unintended adverse effect on quality or appropriateness of care. In Australia it is claimed that the fee schedule encourages excessive appendectomies and tonsillectomies. In Great Britain the original scales for dentists (who unlike specialists and general practitioners are paid on a fee-for-service basis) placed a premium on extractions to the disadvantage of preventive services.

But as against these risks governmental participation in, or operation of, health services has two important advantages over private arrangements, namely, visibility and the existence of an authority that can be held responsible for shortcomings and has power to take remedial action. This advantage is the greater the more nearly universal is the coverage of the public programs. The most impressive feature of the British experience since 1948 has been the extent to which shortcomings of the medical services as they affect the patient and the quality of care have been brought into the open and made the subject of public inquiry and remedial efforts.[24]

Under private arrangements for the supply and financing of health services, many of these shortcomings exist but either they are not brought to light or may be concentrated on "the poor" and disregarded; or, if known, there is no authority in a position to take remedial action.

○ Governmental influence on the organization of the health services. With the exception of a country operating a national health service such as Great Britain, governments appear to have done relatively little to effect an orderly and convenient organization of services. This is probably due to three factors. First, short of compulsion or direct operation by government, it has not proved possible to ensure that all organized groups will subordinate their own interests in perpetuating the status quo, to conform to the requirements of some over-all national plan (especially when it might mean ceding some responsibilities to others or even, at the extreme, going out of business). Second, an over-all plan may well indicate the need for certain services or agencies that are unlikely to be made available except by direct public provision. Third, in some areas there does not appear to be any agreement among professionals as to the nature of the ideal organization. What, for example, should be the role of the general hospital in the total structure of health services? Is group (as opposed to solo) practice the ideal to be sought? And what is to be its nature? What ought to be the relationship of the general practitioner to the hospital? What, ideally, is the role and nature of "community health services," and what should be their relationship to hospitals on the one hand, and the general practitioner's services on the other? Here is another area where the nonmedical social planner lacks authoritative guidance from the health professions.

Even Great Britain has not succeeded in resolving many of these organizational problems. The decision to nationalize the hospitals and to divide the country into hospital regions, each containing one or more teaching hospitals and each with a Regional Hospital Board responsible for planning an integrated series of institutions for its own region, for the preparation of budgets, and for the administration of the funds granted by the government, has indeed made possible a comprehensive and rational organization of hospital services (even though, as pointed out above, hospital construction has fallen short of indicated needs[25]). Even here, the existence of a largely independently administered system of teaching hospitals has created some problems. But the decision (in deference to professional wishes and historical traditions) to organize, on separate bases, the general practitioner services (including dental and ophthalmic services) and certain local health services (largely of a preventive character, but including also ambulance services, health visiting district nursing, home helps, domiciliary midwifery, and prenatal clinics), has created problems of coordination. The problems are likely to become more acute because Britain, too, has become increasingly committed to the doctrine of "getting the patient back into the community." It is far from clear whether all local authorities will be willing or able (even with subsidies from the central government) to develop all the needed community facilities and services. Nor, despite an earlier commitment, has any real progress been made in the development of local health centers to bring together, in one building, preventive, general practitioner, and certain diagnostic services. Financial restrictions and a growing loss of enthusiasm on the part of the medical profession for this type of organization appear largely to account for declining interest in the local health center and the substitution of measures to encourage group practice (such as governmental loans for buildings or office accommodation).

Another example of an effort by government to encourage the development of a more rational structure of health services is represented by the federal government's offer of grants-in-aid to encourage community assessment of needs and development of plans to meet them. Thus the Hill-Burton program of subsidies for hospital construction required as a condition of eligibility that states prepare a plan of hospital needs. The Medical Facilities Survey and Construction Act of 1956 provides grants for, *inter alia,* surveying the needs for treatment centers, certain specialized hospitals, rehabilitation centers, and nursing homes. A series of Federal Mental Health Acts (the most recent of which deals specifically with mental retardation) provide funds to stimulate state (and sometimes community) assessment of, and planning for, needs in this area. Occasionally the federal government itself carries out such planning activities, the most notable example probably being the creation of the Joint Commission on Mental Illness and Health in 1955 that issued an influential report in 1960.[26]

## Problems Related to the Economical Use of Social Resources

The consumer as a member of a society in which resources are limited in relation to needs and wants has an interest in seeing that

70

adequate health care is made available in a way that makes minimum demands on total economic resources. Unnecessary utilization of personnel, health institutions, or supplies (such as drugs) means that a corresponding volume of resources is not available to meet other needs.

## The Role of the Private Sector

*The consumer.* In the normal competitive private enterprise market, control is exercised by individual income receivers who are presumed to buy in the cheapest market. They select from among competing producers those who are so efficient that they can offer their wares at minimum cost (i.e., they make minimum demands on available resources in order to produce what they have to sell).

For the provision of health services this kind of control is much less effective; indeed, current arrangements for the supply and financing of health services would seem rather to foster overuse of resources. The lack of technical knowledge on the part of the consumer, as in regard to quality, puts him at a disadvantage in knowing how much of any kind or type of treatment is absolutely essential (e.g., how many drugs, diagnostic tests, x-rays, and the like, are necessary—how long a stay in hospital is indicated) for the efficient treatment of any complaint.

The limited extent of insurance covering outpatient, diagnostic, and other services to other than hospital inmates or the costs of care in institutions less economically costly than hospitals, such as nursing homes, chronic disease facilities, and the like, coupled with the sheer nonavailability of such less expensive institutions in many areas, tends inevitably to foster overuse of the facility for which insurance is available. Similarly, the lack of appropriately organized community services to continue necessary treatment of the discharged patient is generally agreed to result in longer (and costlier) hospital stays than are essential (though here a caveat should be interposed, for too little is known of the actual cost of a truly adequate supply of community-based medical and ancillary services needed to assist the patient and the family to whom he returns). Again, it has been held that the fear of damage suits (or high insurance rates) has encouraged the proliferation of diagnostic tests that cause so much complaint among consumers.

A further difficulty arises because the market for health services is not competitive. Generally, in the field of institutional care, facilities are not constructed in response to the prospects of profit, and suppliers do not compete with each other on a price (i.e., efficiency) basis. Hospitals may be constructed or expanded because of civic pride or because of the availability of philanthropic funds. Excess bed capacity may be reflected in higher charges for occupied beds, but the consumer has no way of knowing how far the higher price is due to this factor or to other, more economically justified, costs. The efficiency of operation of, e.g., hospitals is not subject to the normal control of inefficiency, whereby the inefficient operator is driven out of business. Only recently, as organized purchasers of hospital services have begun to fear that hospital insurance may be "priced out of the market," have probing questions been raised about the economic operation of hospitals, and these have come from public officials evaluating proposed premium increases.

To the extent that overuse of resources is attributable to the behavior of consumers, organized sellers of insurance can exercise some control on rising quantity and cost by restricting the forms or duration of care against the costs of which they will insure or by introducing "deductibles" and "coinsurance." The former policy may, however, adversely affect total treatment while both limit the extent to which insurance helps the consumer with his financial problem.

*The medical profession.* Heavy reliance appears to be placed on the medical profession to control excessive utilization of scarce resources, but it is doubtful whether any profession, especially in the health services, can be expected to carry this responsibility.

First, the physician is subject to pressures from his patient that may be difficult to resist. Reference has already been made to the overuse of hospitals when hospitalization is the only way in which a patient can be reimbursed for some medical procedures. All systems, public and private, have encountered problems of overuse of pharmaceuticals, or of the use of more expensive proprietary drugs than is necessary. While part of this is undoubtedly attributable to the professional convenience of the doctor, no small part of it appears to stem from pressure from patients.

Second, all professions, including the medical, appear to suffer from a chronic occupational disease that takes two forms: one, an unwillingness to recognize the fact that there are other claims on national resources, and that what is devoted to health services is taken away from some other use; and two, an overestimation of the degree of training essential to the proper performance of all "medical acts." The first results in an insistence on optimum conditions (equipment, premises, time allowances, etc.) believed favorable to what is currently regarded as high quality practice. The second leads to a reluctance to relinquish to less highly trained workers certain types of services or procedures once the exclusive prerogative of the profession. Both lead to unnecessary use of resources to achieve a given result.

Third, all professions appear to be characterized by what I have elsewhere termed "professional myopia": they tend to diagnose all problems in terms of the kind of expertise they are uniquely equipped to provide. Yet some "health" or "medical" problems may require for their solution measures other than "medical treatment," and to continue to deal with them solely by calling for the services of more expensively trained medical personnel involves a waste of economic resources. Illustrations of this kind of myopia abound. The reluctance with which the medical profession accepted the psychic element in illness is one. The relative lack of involvement of the medical profession in efforts to secure better housing, or more adequate income for the poor—both of which have a direct bearing on the health of individuals—is another. And once again the parallel can be drawn with social work. As social workers have become more professionally self-conscious and have identified professionalism with an ability to improve the functioning of the individual they have tended to diagnose most social problems as calling for more social workers rather than for environmental change that might relieve the pressures on individuals and diminish the need for supportive services from social workers.

Fourth, avoidance of excessive use of economic resources requires the cooperation of many professional groups, of which the medical profession is only one, albeit the one most strategically placed.

### The Role of Government

Although, as previously stated, governments have tended to concentrate on the problem of the financial barrier to receipt of health services, and to avoid so far as possible involvement in the structure and organization of these services, they have inevitably been concerned with the effective use of resources as this reflects itself in the cost of the program.

For from this point of view public responsibility for financing part of or all health services has the overwhelming advantages of visibility and accountability. The costs are immediately apparent and, because they must be covered by taxation (or contributions in social insurance systems), the administrators must justify their budgets and defend the efficiency of their operations to the reluctant taxpayers.

Where, as in the British Health Service, government operates its own institutions, the pressures from taxpayers to keep costs down has led to a series of investigations into the efficiency of operation of hospitals, etc., and some notable reforms.[27] But the great advantage in terms of economizing resources, of the nationalization of hospitals both voluntary and those operated by local government, was the possibility offered, and taken, of restructuring the whole set of institutions so as to avoid wasteful deployment of resources. This was probably the one truly revolutionary feature of the British Health Service.

Short of power to compel reorganization (including the suppression of unneeded or overlapping facilities) the public health insurance administration can exercise only the powers of a large-scale buyer, although these may be considerable. In negotiating reimbursement terms with hospitals or other privately operated institutions it is in an especially good position to influence the efficiency of operation (1) because the business it has to confer is so large; (2) because it will have dealings with so many different institutions that comparative analyses can be made and concepts of "normal" costs can be developed; and (3) because, as part of its accountability responsibilities, it can make public reports on the causes, as it sees them, of the high costs of the health service.

The existence of a large-scale consumer-oriented organization purchasing health services does not, of course, ensure that service will be rendered at minimum cost. But it introduces an element of "countervailing" power into a situation characterized by a high degree of monopoly on the part of sellers of service. In some cases the organization, as a large-scale user of supplies, may undertake direct production (e.g., of drugs) although the threat to do so is often sufficient to cause private producers to lower prices.

Where government is the buyer of limited services only, or of complete service for a limited group, its power to insist on economical operation of the institutions from which service is purchased is of course much less.

Insofar as wasteful use of resources is attributable to consumer misuse (excessive calls on physicians' time, overutilization of drugs, carelessness in the use of appliances), governments have made use of some of the same controls as are used by private insurance. Copayment in the form of a requirement to make some minimum payment for prescriptions or appliances in service programs and deductibles and coinsurance in the reimbursement systems are quite extensively used although, as pointed out earlier, they may create financial barriers to needed services.

## The Challenge to the Medical Profession

The growing involvement of government in health services admittedly imposes new demands on the medical profession. For the experience of all countries demonstrates that the interests of the profession (whether in regard to remuneration, or conditions of employment and practice, or the provision of an institutional or

74

organizational structure conducive to the rendering of high-quality service) are likely to be assured only when the profession itself participates actively in the program, over and above providing service for stipulated payments. It means involvement in both policy formation and administration. There is, indeed, scarcely any aspect of the functioning of a comprehensive governmental program that does not call for the active participation of representatives of the health professions.[28]

This would be a relatively new role for medical men in the United States, and it is one that makes special demands on its more distinguished members. More than any other factor it is the willingness or unwillingness of the profession to assume these new responsibilities that will determine whether or not the increasing role of government in the health services will result not only in wider availability but also in improved service.

## Notes

1. Merriam, IC: Social welfare expenditures. *Social Security Bulletin*, XXVI, 11 (November, 1963) *passim*. For later figures see Rice, DP and Cooper, BS: National health expenditures, 1929-70. *Social Security Bulletin*, Vol XXXIV, No 1, (January 1971); 3-18.

1a. Merriam, loc cit, 11. It should be noted that these figures exclude for government support of such activities as research training or capital outlays for research facilities, and, for the private sector, the research expenditures by pharmaceutical, medical supply and medical electronic industries because their cost is presumably included in the price of the product.

2. Reed, LS and Rice, DP: Private consumer expenditures for medical care and voluntary health insurance. *Social Security Bulletin*, Vol XXVI, No 12 (December 1963), 7-8.

3. *Ibid*, 11.

4. For an analysis of coverage by level of family income and size of family, see Lawrence PS, Fuchsberg R: Medical care and family income. *Indicators* (May 1964).

5. Bureau of Labor Statistics study, cited in *Poverty in the United States*, House of Representatives Committee on Education and Labor, HR Committee Print, Washington, DC, 1964, 212.

6. In 1962 insurance companies accounted for 52.4% of total income of these plans and 47.8% of all benefit expenditures. The corresponding proportions in 1948 were 48.8% and 37.6%. Reed, Rice, *op cit*, 9.

7. *Ibid.*, 11.

8. Average vendor payments per recipient for medical care to old age assistance recipients in December, 1963, ranged from $73.46 in Wisconsin and $69.64 in Minnesota to $0.46 in Montana and $1.48 in Mississippi, the national average being $15.44. Among the states that have adopted programs of medical assistance for the aged, average expenditure per recipient in the same month ranged from $439.00 in Illinois and $357.12 in Vermont to $21.58 in Kentucky and $21.90 in West Virginia, the average being $201.20. US Department of Health, Education and Welfare: Program and operating statistics. *Welfare in Review*, 1964.

9. For a concise account of the Australian system see Fox T: The Antipodes: Private practice publicly supported. *Lancet*, April 20 and 27, 1963, 875-879, 983-993. Alberta in 1963 also introduced a system of subsidies toward the

purchase of comprehensive medical benefits payable, however, on the basis of an income test.

10. Volume and cost of sickness benefits in cash and kind. *Bulletin of the International Social Security Association,* XVI (March-April, 1963), 112-115.

11. *Royal Commission on Health Services,* Vol 1. Government of Canada, Ottawa, Duhamel, 1964.

12. Thus in France, in the general scheme, where in principle the beneficiary is expected to pay 20% of total expenses (except for long-duration sicknesses and certain expensive treatments) the beneficiaries' actual share is closer to 50% because of the difference between the reimbursement tariff and the actual fees charged by doctors, dentists, and midwives. In Norway the system reimburses 60 to 65% of the first and second visit to a physician, within the limits set by an official tariff. For severe illnesses 70% is reimbursed. In Sweden 75% of the physician's fee up to the legal tariff is reimbursed, while 50% of the cost of drugs in excess of a minimum sum are reimbursed. There is some evidence that because of the shortage of supply of physicians it is possible for practitioners to charge in excess of the tariff, and it has been estimated that in Stockholm in 1958 the insurance system reimbursements amounted to only about 60% of the charges. *Sickness Insurance: National Monographs.* Geneva, International Social Security Association, 1956, *passim.*

13. See also Abel-Smith B: Major patterns of financing and organization of medical care in countries other than the United States. *Bulletin of the New York Academy of Medicine,* XL, 1964, 540-59. For an account of the arrangements in different countries, see Hogarth J: *The Payment of the General Practitioner,* Oxford, Pergamon, 1963; Glasser W: *Paying the Doctor—Systems of Remuneration and Their Effects,* (Baltimore: Johns Hopkins Press) 1970.

14. *Relations between Social Security Institutions and the Medical Profession,* Geneva, International Social Security Association, 1953; *Sickness Insurance: National Monographs, loc cit.*

15. The various viewpoints and supporting evidence are summarized in Chapter 5 of Harris S: *The Economics of American Medicine.* New York, Macmillan, 1964. The physician ratio in the United States was reported by the Bane Committee as being 132.7 per 100,000 population in 1959. For the same year, the World Health Organization of the United Nations, using as its measure population per physician reported a somewhat lower ratio, namely 790 population per physician (Bane figure would yield 754). Comparable figures for other countries (population per physician ratio) in 1959 were, New Zealand 700, Germany 730, Australia 860, Norway 900, Canada 920, England and Wales 960, Sweden 1,100, Finland 1,600 (Annual Epidemiological and Vital Statistics, Geneva, V 40, 1959, passim). For a later analysis, not available when this paper was written, see Fein R: *The Doctor Shortage: an Economic Diagnosis.* Washington, DC, The Brookings Institution, 1967.

16. In 1951 in the 10 states with lowest per capita income the ratio of physicians per 100,000 population was 83; in the 10 highest income states it was 135. There were sharp regional variations in the distribution of nonfederal physicians (from 164.1 per 100,000 civilian population in New England to 85.1 in the East South Central) and even sharper differences among states (from 287.3 in the District of Columbia or 185.3 in New York to 69.2 in Mississippi and 71.7 in Alabama). As Harris (p. 161) shows, these relative scarcities were reflected in incomes; despite the lower per capita income in the Southeastern states general practitioners' incomes averaged higher (by $1510) than those of general practitioners in the wealthier Northeastern states, and full-time specialists in these poor states earned more than the U.S. average, indeed more than specialists in any region except the Northwest. Harris, *op cit,* 116, 161.

17. *Ibid,* Table 1, p 117.

18. Lindsey A: *Socialised Medicine in England and Wales: The National Health Service, 1948-1961.* Chapel Hill, University of North Carolina Press, 1962, Chapter 6 and *passim.*

19. Evang K et al: *Medical Care and Family Security.* Englewood Cliffs, NJ, Prentice Hall, 1963, p 78.

20. A small number of unions directly operate union health centers that may offer limited or extensive services. The United Auto Workers is the most noteworthy example of a consumer-oriented group endeavoring to grapple with problems of organization, but hitherto its success has been limited. The Somers'

conclusion seems inescapable: "As of the present, it is clear that the medical consumers' new spokesman—the health and welfare plans—have been too contradictory and inconsistent to affect the organization of medical care to the extent that their numerical and financial strength might suggest." Somers H, Somers A: *Doctors, Patients and Health Insurance.* Washington, DC, The Brookings Institution, 1961, 236, Chapter 17.

21. *Ibid,* Chapter 5.

22. Rogers ES: Delegation and control in government-hospital relationships. *Hospital Administration,* 1963, 18-29.

23. In the dental service in Britain, which operates on a fee-for-service basis, the more expensive and complicated operations (one fifth of the total) require the approval of a dental estimates board, seven of whose nine members are dentists. Over the years the list of procedures requiring approval has been somewhat shortened, although not to the full extent desired by the British Dental Association.

24. Lindsey, *op cit,* is replete with illustrations of this point.

25. *Ibid,* Chapters 10 and 11.

26. *Action for Mental Health: Final Report of the Joint Commission on Mental Health.* New York, Basic Books, 1961.

27. Lindsey, *op cit,* Chapters 10 and 11.

28. For an elaboration of this point see below, Chapters 4 and 6.

# 4

# Alternative Financing and Delivery Systems

In many countries public action has removed the costs of necessary medical care from three categories of individuals (and sometimes their families). These three groups are military forces and veterans; persons whose disability arises out of, and in connection with, their employment; and persons whose resources are so meager that they have been found eligible for receipt of income from public assistance. By 1955 most countries with substantial income security systems, other than the United States, had also developed other public programs whereby workers, and sometimes all citizens, receive medical care free, or at reduced cost, unaccompanied by any requirement to undergo a test of need.

These programs have taken three major forms: public subsidies to voluntary insurance organizations, most usually mutual benefit societies or clubs, or trade unions organized to provide medical care for their members; compulsory social insurance systems, whereby workers who have paid the necessary number of contributions are entitled to secure all, or specified types, of medical care free or at reduced cost; and national health systems under which medical care (of all or specified types) becomes a free commodity, like roads or public education, which is supplied by the state.[1]

## The Three Most Common Systems

Because the decision to add the costs of medical care to the range of risks for which public responsibility is accepted implies a knowledge of alternative ways of financing and organizing the supply of medical care,

From Chapter 8, Burns E.M.: *Social Security and Public Policy.* Copyright ©1956 by McGraw-Hill, Inc. Used with permission of McGraw-Hill Book Company.

the nature of the three most common forms of public program calls for description.

The method of subsidizing voluntary health insurance plans is the oldest but is also the one which has been least favored in recent years, although many proposals for the adoption of this method have been made in the United States. Under this system, as it has developed in a number of European countries, certain types of nonprofit health insurance plans receive a subsidy from public funds provided they meet specified conditions which usually relate to membership, minimum benefits to be provided, and financial stability. No country has achieved one hundred percent coverage of the population, or even of all workers, by this method, for the obvious reason that the incomes of some persons are too small to permit them to pay the premiums even when lowered by the public subsidy, while, so long as membership is voluntary, there are always some people who could afford the premiums but who refuse to insure. Furthermore, experience has shown that in the effort to reduce premiums so as to make such insurance available to lower-income groups, public subsidies have increased in proportion to income from contributions or premiums, and with this increasing subsidization has gone, understandably enough, an increase in public control. Inevitably at some point the question has been raised whether such a system differs in any major respect from a wholly public program, except in the complexity of its organization. The urge to substitute a wholly public program has been strengthened by the fact that under the system of subsidized voluntary plans, levels of service vary not only with the efficiency of management of the individual funds but also with the character of their membership and notably its occupational composition and economic level and its geographical location. Hence the general tendency has been either to introduce indirect methods of compulsion[2] or to transform the system into one of the other two types of public medical care program.

Systems of compulsory health insurance are in general form closely similar to compulsory social insurance plans for income security. Certain categories of persons (either workers and the self-employed or workers and their employers) are required to pay contributions (or taxes) on the basis of which an insured worker is entitled to benefits. But the benefit takes the form either, as in Germany or the earlier British health insurance system, for example, of free access to certa defined types of medical services, or, as in the French and other systems, of indemnifying the patient for all, or a part, of the fees he has paid the doctor, hospital, or pharmacist. The insured person usually has free choice of doctor or at least of those doctors who have indicated their willingness to practice under the system. Sometimes the insurance funds own their own hospitals and clinics, but more usually service is supplied by other public or private health agencies, who are reimbursed directly or via the patient from the insurance funds.

Under a public medical service the defined categories of persons who are eligible obtain medical care as needed from physicians and other medical personnel and receive treatment in institutions which are financed by public funds and are usually publicly owned and operated. The suppliers of professional services may be remunerated in a variety of ways which are often identical with those found in compulsory health insurance systems. However, usually no direct financial transactions occur between the recipient and the donor of medical care. For the persons covered, who in some countries, such as Great Britain, may be the whole population, the system is in all respects similar in operation to the public educational service, for access to the service is conditional neither on the passage of a test of need or income nor on the prior payment of contributions.

The different methods whereby government has sought to remove the burden of costs of medical care from individuals and families have many similarities but also some fundamental differences. The extent of the medical services offered, or reimbursable, for example, can be wide or narrow under any method. Some health insurance systems offer only a limited range of care. The British health insurance system, for example, was essentially a general-practitioner service. Other types of medical care were available, if at all, only as additional benefits offered by those approved Societies (the administrative bodies), which by reason of good management or low incidence of illness among their members were in an unusually favorable financial position. Other schemes, such as the French and some other European systems, have been more ambitious, offering a complete range of medical services including specialist service, hospitalization, dental care, and rehabilitation.

On the other hand, while some national health services, such as the British, remove from the patient the costs of an almost unlimited variety and extent of medical care, there are others that offer a very narrow range of care. In the American states, for example, a public medical and dental service for the inspection of all school children is very common, but this public service does not typically extend to the treatment of all children found by such inspection to be in need of remedial care. Similarly, some countries provide for complete health service under public auspices for sufferers from tuberculosis although they do not take a similar responsibility for other types of illness.

Similarly under any type of system the range of persons covered may be wide or narrow. There are some public medical service programs that are limited to defined categories of people. Medical and health care for veterans as provided in the United States and elsewhere is an example of a wholly public medical care program of this type. On the other hand, some national health services, such as those of Great Britain and New Zealand, cover the entire population. Some compulsory health insurance systems (such as the British between 1911 and 1948) have provided care only for the covered worker and make no provision for the medical needs of the dependent family, while others (such as the French and German systems) cover the family as well. Some insurance systems are limited to certain categories of wage earners, while others have covered almost an entire population, though it would admittedly be difficult to cover everyone if eligibility for the service is conditional upon the prior payment of contributions by the sick individual or on his behalf. Even here, however, universal coverage could be secured on an insurance basis if some other public authority, e.g., a public assistance agency, were prepared to pay the premiums for such persons. From this point of view, a public medical service would merely be a less complicated method of achieving universal coverage.

Nor is there a major difference between the various systems in the extent to which they involve the government in negotiations with the appropriate professions regarding the terms of remuneration. Under any system, if the burdens of medical costs are to be effectively removed from the patient, or their incidence is to be substantially lightened, the public authorities become concerned with the methods of remuneration and the nature of the charges of the medical profession. This is obvious under a public medical service. Here the government must be able to attract and retain the services of such medical personnel as are needed to provide the promised medical benefits to the eligible population. Whatever the method of remuneration adopted (and, as will be shown below, a variety of methods including salary, fee-for-service, and the capitation system is available), the economic return to the members of the professions concerned must prove sufficiently attractive to assure the desired supply. But under an indemnity system, too, a government becomes involved in the economics of the medical profession. For the amount of the indemnity must clearly be related to the normal charges of the physician. If, as has been the case in New Zealand, for example, the government scheme reimburses the patient by a fixed payment for each visit of the doctor but leaves the medical man free to charge a total fee as much above this sum as he thinks the traffic will bear, the only effect of such a plan may be to offer an income guarantee to all doctors, and the patient may still find himself burdened with a heavy cost. If there is then pressure on the government to raise the level of the indemnity, the total costs of the service may vastly increase and give rise to pressure on both government and the medical profession to reach some agreement about acceptable charges. Such a settlement might take the form of drawing up approved schedules for charges for different types of service or an agreement on the part of the profession to accept the public indemnity in full settlement of their bill to the patient, in which case the amount of the indemnity becomes a vital issue. In either event, government becomes involved in problems of the proper remuneration of a profession.[3]

Finally, as we have seen, not even the subsidized voluntary insurance schemes can eliminate the necessity for standard setting by government, although here the degree of public intervention in the rendering of service is admittedly less than under a compulsory health insurance system and very much less than under a public medical service.

It is doubtful, too, whether the distinction between compulsory health insurance and a public medical or health service lies in the form in which the patient receives his benefit, that is to say whether the plan offers merely an indemnification of all or part of medical costs incurred, or provides benefits in the form of direct medical services. The indemnity system, as we have seen, occurs in voluntary health insurance systems, where it is very usual, in compulsory health insurance systems, and in at least one national health service (that of New Zealand). While changing to the minimum degree the basis of organizing and financing medical care, it has been rejected by many systems for the reasons that:

> The system of direct provision of benefits is the more appropriate system where the full cost, with few exceptions, is borne by the state. It is more convenient for the patient, to the professions involved, to the hospitals and other institutions, and is simpler administratively. It does not require the patient to have money available before seeking treatment and avoids any financial barrier between patient and treatment.[4]

On the other hand, the strength of the organized professions has ensured its retention in many systems, of which the French and New Zealand systems are notable examples. For to the professions, the indemnity system serves as a guarantee of minimum income since it assures the collection of fees up to the amount of the public reimbursement, and where physicians have been able successfully to charge fees over and above the amount reimbursed, the system offers them every advantage. For the community, however, the indemnity system merely increases the effective demand for medical care but offers no guarantee either that there will be any expansion of preventive health services or even that the supply of personnel and facilities will be expanded in response to the increased demand for curative services. At least one country has rejected the indemnity system in favor of direct provision of service by the insurance funds on the ground that the latter is more economical.[5]

The major differences between the various public systems hitherto developed would seem to relate to two characteristics: whether the right to benefit is or is not conditional upon the prior payment of a specified number of contributions; and whether government, in developing the program, accepts responsibility for assuring the availability of adequate personnel and facilities for meeting all types of health needs.

The presence or absence of a contributory requirement as a condition of eligibility is a very important differentiating characteristic of the nonmeans test public systems. Under a public medical service, the right of the patient to receive services (or occasionally reimbursement) is not, as it is under health insurance systems, dependent on the prior payment of contributions, or for that matter on any other test.[6] This overcomes one of the disadvantages of compulsory health insurance, namely that the system of requiring prior contributions as a condition of eligibility inevitably bars some individuals from access to the service. While a case may be made for this kind of barrier in income security programs, no public interest can be invoked for denying medical care and rehabilitation to persons in need of such services. At the same time, national health systems differ from systems of public medical care available under public assistance laws in that eligibility is not conditional upon passing a needs test.

In the second place, the systems differ according to the range and scope of the responsibilities accepted by the government. Under a public medical service the government not only removes all or part of the cost of medical care from those covered by the plan but also itself accepts responsibility for ensuring a supply of services and facilities to the extent called for by the health needs of the eligible group. Thus in the veterans' health program in the United States it is the federal government which builds hospitals and other facilities, which hires the needed medical personnel (by salary or other arrangements), and which sets the standards of service. Similarly, in Great Britain, where in 1946 the people authorized their government "to promote the establishment . . . of a comprehensive health service designed to secure the improvement in the physical and mental health of the people . . . and the prevention, diagnosis and treatment of illness," it was inevitable that the relevant act should add "and to provide, or secure the effective provision, of services in accordance with the foregoing provisions." Since in Britain the coverage of the service is universal and embraces all kinds of health service, this has meant in fact that the government is held responsible for assuring that adequate personnel and facilities are available everywhere, that acceptable standards of service are rendered, that appropriate provision is made for research and training, and that these requirements are met with a maximum of economy.

This is perhaps the feature of a national health service that distinguishes it most sharply from an indemnity health insurance system, however wide the scope and coverage of the latter. In the typical health insurance plan all the government does, in effect, is to remove the economic barrier to access to whatever medical services of the defined types may be available. If the patient cannot find a hospital in his community, that is no concern of the program. If certain necessary specialists are not available, the sick person has no complaint against the government, which offers only to meet his costs if he can find a specialist to care for him. If there are too few doctors in his community, or if the general level of professional practice is low, this too is no responsibility of the government. Under a public medical service, however, all these become matters for which government has accepted responsibility and for which it is held accountable.

## Problems Peculiar to Public Medical Services

A government administering a public medical service, particularly if its scope is wide, thus faces a number of difficult problems, additional to those which it has in common with compulsory health insurance systems and which will be discussed in the following section. First, and most obvious of these, is the necessity of finding an acceptable compromise between the demand of the citizens for a high-grade medical and health service and their reluctance to devote to this purpose the necessary proportion of the national income.[7] It does not yet seem possible to say whether or not in the long run a comprehensive national health service requires a nation to devote a larger proportion of the national income than hitherto to health maintenance and promotion. It is true that, to some extent, a public medical service (or for that matter a compulsory health insurance system) represents merely another way of paying for health services (i.e., by averaging costs over the entire covered group and paying them through insurance contributions or taxes). But the experience of all countries that have instituted such measures indicates that when first enacted, the demands on medical facilities (human and institutional) increase very greatly once the economic barrier to their use is removed, and if these are to be met, a larger share of the national income must be devoted to health services.

To some extent this increased demand for medical service is to be expected and even hoped for, since one of the objects of such a program is to ensure that people get medical care as and when they need it, regardless of their ability to pay. But against this initial and often heavy demand for the allocation of increased resources to meet medical needs must be set the possibility that early treatment in cases now too often allowed to run their course will, in time, reduce the need for much care previously given. It has also been held that greater emphasis on preventive medicine will in the long run tend to reduce the proportion of the national income devoted to curative services.[8]

It remains to be seen whether these influences will offset the general upward trend in the costs of medical care due to scientific developments in medicine itself and to the consumer's demand for a higher standard of health.[9]

In the short run, however, there is no doubt that governments instituting such systems are under great pressure to devote larger resources to the service, because of the heavy backlog of previously unmet needs. In a very rich country this may present no insuperable difficulties. But the securing of a proper balance between the health services and other services which make demands upon the taxpayer's income has been an acute problem in Great Britain, which instituted the National Health Service at the very moment when the nation faced the necessity of making good from limited national resources the attritions and obsolescences in its capital equipment occasioned by World War II.

In view of the heavy and mounting costs of high standard medical care and the inadequacy of medical personnel and facilities in relation to accumulated needs in the initial stages of such programs, it is not surprising that those responsible for the development and administration of comprehensive health services have to make difficult choices, for priorities must be established, and these always expose the administrator to pressures from interested groups and to criticism when a choice has been made. Thus the British government has been criticized by some members of the medical profession and others for regarding the construction of health centers as a postponable item during the first years of the program, and the hospital authorities have constantly complained that inadequate funds have been granted for essential improvements and construction. Nor is it always easy to implement the priorities decided upon.[10]

In any case, if the disproportion is very great between needs, augmented by a substantial backlog, and medical resources, an immediate lowering of the standards of care is likely to result. For if the price of medical service is reduced to zero or almost zero, it will then be necessary to spread these supplies very thin over all who wish to make use of them. Some hold that even so, it is arguable whether this method of rationing resources that are inadequate for total health needs is any worse than the previous system of rationing them, i.e., by the price system, whereby some are able to buy all the medical care they need, while others, because of limited incomes, go short. However poor the standard of care under the public program, it may well be an improvement over that previously received by those who formerly went short or who necessarily judge standards of quality by the service customarily received by the poor rather than by the rich.

Inevitably, therefore, any socialization of the costs of medical care, however achieved, brings to the fore the problem of adequacy of facilities and personnel. Some countries, such as Canada, have decided that before adopting even a health insurance system steps must be taken to increase the supply, and improve the geographical distribution, of medical facilities and personnel, and public funds are currently being used for that purpose. Others, such as Great Britain, have first instituted a free health service and then grappled with the problem of supplies. Which course is preferable, assuming the existence of a desire for public action, would seem to depend upon which one would most speedily bring supply in relation to demand. A public and a medical profession that were prepared to accept some temporary inadequacies but to continue to press for expanded supplies might find the British sequence preferable to the Canadian. Where, however, there is a hostile medical profession or a public poorly informed as to the underlying facts, the lowering of service or even failure of the plan to make good on all kinds of care promised in the early years until supplies catch up with demand might endanger the continuation of the service since it would permit the medical profession to claim that all their worst fears were realized.

Almost inevitably, too, a government caught between the pressure of the consumer for more or higher standards of service and the resistance of the taxpayer to further levies on his income tends to seek ways and means of cutting costs, and these efforts often bring it into conflict with the suppliers of the service. Far too little is known about the effect of these efforts to keep costs to a minimum. On the one hand, it has to be admitted that all professional groups tend to set their requirements for necessary equipment and facilities by reference to criteria which emphasize rather the attainment of the highest possible professional standards than the economic cost of meeting these requirements. They also tend to resist the allocation to auxiliary personnel of functions once peculiar to the fully trained practitioner. On the other hand, unless the lay administrator succeeds in working closely and constructively with his medical advisers and unless the profession is willing to cooperate in keeping costs to a realistic minimum, these enforced economies may lead to an undesirable and even an unnecessary lowering of the standards of service.

In the second place, operation of such a service is likely to cause the government to invade some spheres traditionally held to be the preserve of private enterprise or private philanthropy. Thus the necessity of making the most economical and effective use of hospital resources led the British government in 1948 to take over the existing voluntary hospital system, since it could not undertake the costly task of constructing adequate public hospitals for its own clientele, and the country was in no position to afford the unused bed capacity that would have resulted from two competing hospital systems.[11] The need to ensure adequate coverage of the country as a whole by a well-integrated system of essential health facilities (general and special hospitals, clinics, and the like) also pointed to the desirability of combining existing voluntary and public facilities, by compulsion if necessary. Thus the pressures both of economics and of effective planning for adequate service broadened the sphere of public activity.

Similarly, under a public medical service it is impossible for government not to concern itself with the supply and distribution of medical personnel. Quite apart from the difficult problems of estimating future demand for medical personnel, and more particularly avoiding a future surplus in an effort to meet the heavy backlog of demand typically experienced at the inception of national health services, a government which attempts to ensure an adequate and appropriate supply of trained professional medical personnel is likely to come into conflict with the organized professions. For in many cases the monopoly position of the profession and the level of incomes of its members are maintained by a policy of restriction of entry to the medical schools, and it is hardly likely that the profession and the government will hold the same views regarding the need for an increase in the supply of trainees and training facilities.

Most countries are familiar with the problem of the maldistribution of medical personnel, who tend to concentrate in urban and higher income centers, where medical facilities such as hospitals abound, to the neglect of rural and poorer areas. The methods adopted by governments to remedy this situation may well lead to actions which the professions concerned regard as limitations of individual freedom, or at least as undue intervention in matters which have hitherto been regarded as of purely professional concern. Thus, in Britain, one of the bitterest disputes between the medical profession and the government during the formative period of the National Health Service concerned the machinery set up by the government to prevent new doctors practicing under the service from entering areas classified as "overdoctored." Doctors in independent private practice were, of course, free to set up in practice wherever they wished. More recently the evidence suggests that these arrangements are working smoothly and have been generally accepted by the profession. The alternative solution proposed by medical men—that doctors should be attracted to the "under-doctored areas" by the offer of higher rates of remuneration—would have increased the cost of the service. The rejection by the government of this proposal in favor of the device of negative control accompanied by a system of "inducement payments," limited to the first three years of practice in heavily underdoctored areas, illustrates the different considerations that necessarily govern the public authority and the profession in grappling with a common problem.

Thirdly, under a system of public medical care, government cannot evade ultimate responsibility for the quality of medical care in the broadest sense. This involves much more than assuring that the financial and administrative arrangements adopted do not disturb existing patient-doctor relationships or cause a general lowering of the professional standards of the medical personnel, a problem which the national health service has in common with compulsory health insurance systems. It embraces also such questions as whether the system as a whole devotes the proper relative attention to preventive, as contrasted to curative, services; whether adequate provision is made for convalescent or rehabilitative services; whether adequate stimulus is given to research; whether the mental health services are appropriately developed; and the like. These are, of course, not questions that can properly be asked only about a public service; they are in fact often asked in countries which rely almost wholly on private enterprise for the provision of health and medical services. But under a public program, for the first time the facts are a matter of public record, and some one authority is held answerable for failures to reach desired standards for the country as a whole. It might indeed be said that a much higher standard is required of government than of private enterprise in this respect, and the resulting greatly increased vulnerability to criticism may be one of the considerations which have led to some reluctance on the part of governments to select the alternative of the national health or medical service.

## X Problems Common to Compulsory Health Insurance and Public Medical Services

Among the many organizational and administrative problems that are faced alike by health insurance systems and national health or medical services three call for special emphasis, namely the development of appropriate methods of remunerating professional and technical personnel; the development of a plan whose over-all effects will tend to improve rather than lower the standards of medical care; and the invention and operation of devices for avoiding overuse of the service.

### *Methods of Remunerating Professional Personnel*

Both compulsory health insurance systems and national health services have to resolve the problem of devising methods of remunerating professional personnel which will attract and retain an adequate supply of practitioners and which will foster, rather than impede, the rendering of service of high quality. The selection of appropriate methods of remuneration has, in fact, been a major cause of controversy between governments and the professions involved.

A variety of methods has been developed of which the best known are the fee-for-service, payment by salary, and the capitation systems. The fee-for-service system is found, for example, in the French and New Zealand general systems and applies to dental practitioners in Great Britain. Here the insurance fund or the national administration either reimburses the doctor directly in accordance with the services he has rendered or reimburses the patient for all or part of his medical bills. Sometimes it is provided that the attending physician must accept the sum paid by the state in full settlement of his claim. In other cases, he may be allowed to charge what the traffic will bear, over and above the reimbursable sum. As a rule, especially where the public institution pays the patient a percentage of the doctor's bill, detailed schedules of permitted charges are developed by the public authority, usually in consultation with the medical profession.

The fee-for-service system has the advantage of being most similar to

90

that prevailing in private practice and is the one generally favored by medical practitioners. It allows the evaluations of the market place, as expressed by the actions of patients, the widest scope. The popular doctor will have many patients and a larger income than his less popular colleague, and if the judgment of patients reflects a true evaluation of the relative professional skill of the two men, then the fee-for-service system operates to reward efficiency and promotes high standards. This condition is, however, not always satisfied. And on the other hand, the fee-for-service system has several disadvantages. It is highly cumbersome, requiring as it does that doctors and/or patients keep detailed records of the services rendered. It is likely to require the development of elaborate schedules of fees for different types of service, and quite apart from the technical difficulties of this task, the relative money values attached to different services may influence the types of care or treatment given. If, for example, in dentistry, the price set for extractions exceeds that for preventive treatment, some practitioners may be tempted to neglect the latter. In any case, the use of the fee-for-service system is expensive, for it tempts those members of the profession whose desire for economic rewards exceeds their sense of professional responsibility to increase their incomes by unnecessary services. Nor is it easy under a complicated schedule to devise a series of fees that will ensure any desired average level of incomes to the members of the profession.[12]

The method of employing medical personnel on salary avoids some of these difficulties. It is found in the United States in the Veterans Administration and in Sweden and in some Canadian provinces where municipal doctors are employed, and it is utilized in Great Britain for specialists and hospital staffs. It is true that the problem of setting a level of incomes which the profession regards as fair and reasonable and which the public feels is not out of line with the economic rewards of other highly trained professional persons still remains.[13] But it avoids the difficulties of schedule making and the temptations to the weaker members of the profession to allow the nature and frequency of service rendered to be influenced by economic considerations. It also avoids the detailed record keeping characteristic of the fee-for-service system. On the other hand, medical men object that the salaried service offers no rewards to the more skillful or assiduous practitioner. Although this is not wholly true, since salaried services frequently provide for increments according to degrees of skill or experience,[14] there is no doubt that a salaried system would hardly yield the very high incomes that are received by some highly successful practitioners in private practice. There seems less validity in the claim, sometimes made by the spokesmen for organized medicine, at least by implication, that work of high quality cannot be expected if remuneration is on a salaried basis and that only the prospect of high economic rewards stimulates the medical man to his highest professional efforts. However, the administration of a salaried system with rewards for superior performance would necessarily require some members of the profession to sit in judgment upon others. Although this kind of evaluation is common enough in academic circles and is found in other professions that work for salary, it appears to be resisted by the American medical profession, who in the past have demonstrated some reluctance to act as a body in judgment on the competence of a colleague.

The capitation system, which is found in Great Britain and some other countries, endeavors to avoid some of the disadvantages of both fee-for-service and payment by salary. Under this arrangement, which is feasible only for general practice, the patient selects a physician and is enrolled on his panel. The doctor is paid at a fixed annual rate per head for each person on his panel,[15] regardless of whether or not service is required during the year. Typically, a maximum limit is set to the number of patients, or potential patients, who can be enrolled with any doctor.

In support of this system it is urged that it retains some of the incentives of the fee-for-service system. The doctor who is unpopular with his patients will lose them to his competitors, and his panel being smaller, his income will fall. There will thus be an incentive to give good service, and the doctor who works harder because he has more patients will receive a larger income, but there will be no temptation to give unnecessary service. Indeed, it is alleged that under this system it will be to the interest of the doctor by preventive measures to try to keep his patients healthy. Here, too, record keeping for reimbursement purposes is avoided. On the other hand, the determination of appropriate capitation rates presents difficulties. A sum must be fixed such that for the doctor with an average panel and with an average incidence of need for care among his patients and giving service of average quality, the income yielded will again be one that the profession regards as fair and reasonable and the public feels is not too out of line with incomes of persons of a similar degree of training and experience. Furthermore, appropriate allowance has to be made in setting the capitation fee for necessary expenses incurred by the doctor in maintaining his office and equipment.

Where the supply of doctors is limited in relation to the total number of patients, the maximum limits on the size of individual panels may be so high that standards of service suffer. This, however, is not a weakness of the capitation system as such, as has sometimes been argued, but would occur under any method of payment if access to medical service is not restricted by the price system and if supply is short in relation to demand.

## Maintenance of High Standards of Service

The problem of operating a public or a publicly controlled medical care system in such a way as to maintain high standards of service has concerned those who have formulated or administered these measures from the first. Some types of safeguard have been relatively easy to introduce. Thus most systems operating by the mid-century permitted the patient free choice of any doctor admitted to practice under the scheme. As these public programs have come to be well established and accepted by the community and the profession alike, the proportion of all doctors and specialists practicing under the schemes has steadily increased and in some countries (e.g., Great Britain) approaches 100%. It can therefore be argued with some cogency that, since the doctors' probable fees are no longer a consideration, the patients' choice is actually much wider than under a nongovernmental system.

In most systems, too, medical men are free to practice under the public program or not as they wish and to accept or refuse patients who desire their services, subject to normal professional limitations. However, in the case of a national medical service, such as the British, where over 90% of the population has indicated a preference for care through the service, the market for the privately practicing doctor is so narrowed that the average practitioner has in reality little choice but to enter the system.

Medical men have frequently expressed fears than the intervention of government will inevitably interfere with the relationships of doctor and patient and result in a lowering of the quality of care. On the former charge, it has, however, been pointed out that it is by no means certain that patient-doctor relationships, especially where financial transactions are involved, are even now so satisfactory to the patient that the latter would not welcome some changes. And some doctors who have practiced under compulsory health insurance or national health services have held that the removal of direct financial dealings between patient and doctor has made for an improvement of patient-doctor relationships. Many doctors have held, too, that better professional service can be given when the treatment prescribed need no longer be influenced by consideration of the ability of the patient to meet the costs.

The fear that public programs would involve the interposition of third parties between the attending physician and his patient may under certain circumstances be justified, although it is likely to occur only when questions are raised about the appropriateness of treatment given.[16] In reality, most systems prohibit any doctor employed by the fund or agency in a supervisory or controlling capacity from giving treatment to patients. It has been pointed out, too, that the increasing specialization of medical practice has tended to loosen the bonds between the general practitioner and his patients, who in many cases even under private practice receive treatment simultaneously from several medical personnel. This situation, which has been fostered by technical or scientific developments, has indeed strengthened a movement toward group practice, which quite apart from any public medical service, may change the nature of the earlier relationship of doctor and patient, and not necessarily for the worse.

More disturbing to the professional man's normal methods of practice are the controls, embodied in some health insurance or health service systems, whereby prior authority has to be obtained from some committee or official appointed by the administration if certain types of expensive treatment or medicaments are to be prescribed. This is, of course, a real limitation on the complete independence of professional judgment of the individual physician. However, this limitation applies, of course, only to those prescribed under the public system. Such medicaments can always be prescribed and purchased at the patients' own expense. On the other hand, unless a high standard of professional competence and a lively sense of responsibility as to the use of public funds can be relied on in all but a tiny minority of cases, some type of safeguard for the interests of the taxpayer is essential in a system where the public foots the entire bill. The problem of the mounting costs of pharmaceutical expenditures (to be discussed below) indicates that this problem is very real. The practical problem facing those who devise public programs is whether such controlling bodies can be so staffed as to give preponderant representation to professional personnel and yet retain a concern for the interest of the taxpayer.[17]

The effect on standards of service of methods of remunerating physicians has already been touched upon in the preceding section. It would seem that neither capitation nor the salaried service *of necessity* gives rise to poor professional performance unless the sense of professional responsibility is dormant throughout the profession as a whole. And as we have seen, the system of remuneration by fee for service involves no real change for the doctor (except by giving him a guarantee on collections). Many of the unsatisfactory effects on standards of practice that are often charged against the methods of remunerating professional personnel under public insurance or health service systems are in fact rather the consequence of a sudden increase in the demand for medical services, unaccompanied by a corresponding increase in the supply of trained personnel.

The fear that a public service will be unduly vulnerable to political pressures and manipulations has often been expressed by organized medicine in the United States. The experience of other countries, however, seems to suggest that the extent to which this will happen is in large measure within the control of the profession itself. Admittedly, if political pressures (such as influencing appointments or the volume and geographical distribution of physical facilities and the like) are to be resisted, the profession as a whole has to be on the alert, and the leaders who carry weight with the public have to devote time to influencing public opinion and serving on the many advisory and negotiating committees whose existence appears unavoidable if the viewpoint and the interests of the medical profession, scientific as well as economic, are to exert a proper influence.

### Avoiding Overuse of the Service

The experience of all public systems, whether health insurance or public medical service (and indeed of privately organized comprehensive medical care insurance systems), suggests that there is a third problem of major importance, namely the danger of overuse of facilities and medical resources. This overuse may take the form of unnecessary calls upon the time of doctors for trivial complaints; excessive use of hospital facilities where no real need for in-patient care exists; overuse or careless use of medical appliances; or excessively high expenditures on pharmaceuticals. Of these, the last has perhaps been the most dramatic and highly publicized, in the experience of many countries having public programs in recent years,[18] although the rising costs of hospitalization are everywhere causing concern, in public, as in private, systems.

In part, the problem is one for which the medical profession itself is responsible. Unless overprescribing is checked by vigorous pressure from within the ranks of organized medicine, the lay administrators have been forced to adopt controlling measures which have varied from the requirement that the doctor secure prior approval for certain types of costly treatment or drugs to the application of ex post facto administrative controls and impositions of penalties.[19]

In part the problem is attributable to the demands of the consumers of medical care, a commodity on which people in general seem inclined to spend less of their own incomes than is socially desirable but which they will use in great quantities if they get it free. Efforts to check overuse have taken various forms: charging a minimal fee for each visit to the physician or for each unit of service or prescription has been found useful in some systems (e.g., in the British system, for dentures or for renewal of spectacles or other appliances when renewal is occasioned by negligence). Obviously, however, there are limits to the extent to which this control can be used, since a fee that acts as an effective deterrent to frivolous or irresponsible use of the system may deter some low-income groups from using the service in cases of genuine need.[20] Public education has also been relied upon, with varying success.

It is probably true to say that the promotion of responsible use by the citizenry of freely available social services is a major problem faced by those who favor public action to remove the costs of medical care from the average citizen.

## The Determinants of Action

Whether or not a community will decide to invoke the powers of government in the field of medical care, for which population categories and for which types of treatment and care it will develop public programs, and which type of program will be favored will therefore depend upon a number of variables.[21]

The first of these is the degree of dissatisfaction with existing methods of organizing and financing medical care, as judged by the extent of unmet health needs and by the severity of the economic burden of medical costs upon individuals or families. The greater the importance attached by the public to universal access to comprehensive health services of all types, undeterred by any income barrier, the less will be the weight attached to some of the shortcomings of public programs due to failure to solve, or to solve completely, the problems discussed in the preceding sections.

Even when allowance is made for the pricing system customarily practiced by the medical profession, which aims to adjust charges to income, the burden of medical costs, especially when hospital and other care is included,[22] remains heavy for certain families and individuals. There is evidence that many patients, even among those who benefit from reduced rates, resent the type of means-test relationship that is involved in the method of setting fees in private practice. And the other adjustment to the high costs of medical care very commonly found, namely providing through public assistance for the care of needy or medically needy persons, is unpopular and of little help to the vast middle class.

There appears to be agreement that only by some form of insurance can the uneven incidence of medical costs be prevented from overburdening individual families.[23] On the other hand, opinions differ as to whether the average family could afford to pay the premiums necessary to cover the costs of a comprehensive medical care insurance system, and it is generally admitted that the very lowest income groups could hardly buy this kind of protection without seriously depressing their current standard of living. In any case, the American voluntary health insurance plans meet only a part of medical costs, the percentage being estimated at 17.4 in 1952 and 19.5 in 1953.[24] There is also difference of opinion as to how far, even among the groups that are held to be able to afford the premiums, people would be willing, or could be induced, voluntarily to set aside the necessary funds. Some argue that human nature being what it is, nothing short of the compulsion of the tax collector would bring about the desired result.[25]

Existing methods of financing and organizing medical services are also judged by criteria other than their effect on the economic security of individuals and families. Public action in the field of health has thus been stimulated by prevailing dissatisfaction with the over-all results of purely private provision, as measured by mortality and morbidity statistics,[26] the limited extent of constructive services, such as rehabilitative and preventive programs, and the nonavailability of some types of high quality care in certain geographical areas. The more strongly deficiencies of this type are felt by the voters to be unnecessary and undesirable, the greater will be the pressure for public action and action of a character that is more comprehensive than a mere indemnity system.

A second influential force is the attitude to government activity as such: a country like the United States with its strong tradition of free enterprise and fear of government activity may well regard proposals to extend the role of government in the field of medical care with greater reservation than Britain, where a substantial measure of public activity is already accepted and where the citizens as a whole appear to have more confidence in their own powers to control the actions of their governments.

The attitudes and traditions of the medical profession itself are a third major determinant. For governmental programs that aim to meet the costs of specific services rendered by recognized professions, such as education or health, or to supply these services directly obviously involve more complex problems than do those which aim merely to provide alternative income, precisely because they require the enlistment of the full participation and cooperation of the professions involved. To some degree government itself can influence the extent of this cooperation, by providing more or less adequately in its administrative structures and organization for appropriate professional representation in, and control of, those aspects of the program which are properly of professional concern. Experience has shown that in formulating programs too much attention cannot be directed to this matter. On the other hand, it is evident that the effective operation of such plans makes heavy demands on a profession that has hitherto functioned as an uncontrolled and self-governing monopoly, answerable to no one for the over-all effectiveness of its operations. These demands are in essence that the profession should recognize that a public interest attaches to some aspects of its methods of organization and remuneration and should be prepared to subordinate purely professional interests to the wider public welfare.

For the adjustments that the medical profession has to make to the new public policies affecting the organization, remuneration, and supply of medical services are many. The individual practitioner may have to face a change in his methods of remuneration which, while probably increasing the total income of the profession, may significantly alter the total incomes of individual physicians, either upward or downward. He will have to devote more time than formerly to certain civic responsibilities, such as serving as a certifying officer for various social or medical services, from which he has hitherto been mercifully spared. He will have to learn, as the teacher has already learned, how to maintain a good relationship with his clients even though he denies their requests for improper service, supplies, or certifications. The profession as a group may be forced to take stock of the effectiveness of some of its methods of operating since it will be under greater pressure than hitherto to show that results are achieved with a maximum of economy in the use of scarce resources. Above all, the leaders of the profession will find themselves called upon to take time from their specifically professional activities to represent their fellows on the many negotiating, standard-setting, and controlling committees and organizations which are inevitable if the purely professional aspects of the service are to be under medical control and if the economic interests of the practitioners are to be properly protected.

In many countries, and notably perhaps in Great Britain, the physicians and other medical personnel have already demonstrated an ability to accept the implications of the public interest inherent in the functioning of their professions. In the United States, another profession, the teachers, have long adapted themselves to the problems of professional functioning in a publicly controlled service. The willingness of the medical profession in America to come to grips with the problem of how to render professionally acceptable service under a system of organization that is not of their choosing but may be demanded by the public will in the last resort determine not whether such a system will be brought into effect (for no profession can long withstand the demands of the wider community) but rather whether that system, if adopted, will result in a raising or a lowering of the standards of medical care and the general state of health of all the people.

Finally, the nature and viability of public programs concerned with health and medical care will depend upon the character of the citizenry, their capacity to exercise self-restraint in the utilization of freely available goods and services, their preparedness to countenance short-comings when those are attributable to forces beyond the control of the administrator, their determination to initiate action to remedy unjustifiable or inexplicable deficiencies, and their willingness to pay, in taxes, the price of a comprehensive service of high quality.

## Notes

1. For a convenient summary of legislation see Farman, CH: *Health and Maternity Insurance throughout the World, Principal Legislative Provisions.* Reprint of part 8 of Hearings before the House Committee on Interstate and Foreign Commerce, Social Security Administration, Division of Research and Statistics, 1954. For more detail on selected countries, see *Relations between Social Security Institutions and the Medical Profession,* Report IV, Eleventh General Meeting, International Social Security Association, Geneva, 1953 (hereinafter referred to by title only). For developments in the United States, see Michael M. Davis, *Medical Care for Tomorrow,* Harper & Brothers, New York, 1955, *passim.*

2. Thus in Denmark the right to an old-age pension is dependent on membership in a voluntary health insurance fund.

3. A major feature of the operation of the American Emergency Maternity and Infant Care program for meeting the costs of medical care before, during, and after delivery, of the wives of certain grades of servicemen during World War II, for example, was the dispute between the medical profession and the government regarding the latter's insistence that the standard payment to the doctor was to be in full settlement of his claims against the patient.

4. "Memorandum submitted by the Ministry of Pensions and National Insurance, United Kingdom," in *Relations between Social Security Institutions and the Medical Profession,* 247. For a fuller statement of the case against the indemnity system, see the Austrian report in *ibid,* pp 107-108; see also the German reply in *ibid,* 223.

5. See reply of the Austrian Federation of Social Insurance Institutions in *ibid,* 108.

6. The British system even extends this right to foreigners who may find themselves in need of medical care while in the country.

7. See especially Ross, JS: *The National Health Service in Great Britain.* New York, Oxford University Press, 1952, Chapter 32.

8. For an estimate of cost ranges in the United States see Falk, IS: Cost

estimates for national health insurance. *Social Security Bulletin,* August 1949, 4-10. For later estimates see Chapter 9 below.

9. On the influences making for mounting costs of health services regardless of how they are financed, see Roberts, F: *The Cost of Health.* London, Turnstile Press, 1952, Chapters 2-8.

10. Thus despite the statutory priority in the National Health Service Act for dental care for young children and nursing mothers, the administrative arrangements for the supply of this service coupled with the terms of remuneration provided for dentists practicing in the general dental service resulted in a shortage of personnel for the priority services.

11. The necessity for economy in the use of hospital facilities was finally brought home to the country during World War II. Cf. Titmuss, RM: *Problems of Social Policy.* London, HM Stationery Office, 1950, especially Chapter 22-24.

12. Thus the original fee scale devised for dentists practicing under the British National Health Service yielded in fact incomes that were much greater than intended and far out of line with incomes of doctors practicing under the Service. (Ross, *op cit,* pp 232-264).

13. For an interesting discussion of the principles that might be adopted in deciding upon appropriate income levels for professional workers (however remunerated), see the reports of the three committees under the chairmanship of Sir William Spens, which dealt with the problems of remunerating general practitioners, consultants and specialists, and dentists under the British Health Service. (*Reports of the Interdepartmental Committee on the Remuneration of Consultants and Specialists* (1948); *Reports of the Interdepartmental Committee on the Remuneration of General Dental Practitioners* (1948), HM Stationery Office, London.)

14. See for instance the scale adopted in Great Britain for hospital medical and dental staffs (Ross, *op cit,* 151-153).

15. The fee per patient enrolled sometimes varies according to the number of persons on the panel.

16. This type of third party intervention is most likely to occur when the doctor functions as a certifying agent for a cash disability insurance system.

17. For an illuminating discussion of the effects of different types of organizational and other arrangements upon the nature of the service rendered and the impact upon the physician, see *Relations between Social Security Institutions and the Medical Profession, op cit,* especially 9-43.

18. Studies made by the British Ministry of Health and other authorities have shown that mounting pharmaceutical costs are attributable to prescribing porprietary remedies where similar and cheaper nonproprietary medicaments were available, prescribing excessive quantities, too free prescription of new or expensive drugs, and finally some prescriptions for items that are not really drugs. (Cf. Ross, *op cit,* Chapter 21; and *Annual Report of the Ministry of Health,* 1953, London, HM Stationery Office, 1954, *passim.*) For an account of the problem as experienced in other countries, see Tuchman, E: "The Prescription of Medicaments and the Amount Used," in *Reports of the Permanent Committees* I, Medico-Social Committee, International Social Security Association, Geneva, 1954, 22-42.

19. For an account of the administrative controls developed in Great Britain, see *Bulletin of the International Social Security Association,* June-July, 1954, 226-228.

20. However, in countries with an adequately financed and publicly acceptable general assistance program this difficulty can be overcome, as in Great Britain, by permitting those for whom this payment would be a hardship to secure reimbursement from the assistance agency.

21. For the attitudes of different groups in America toward proposals for public action prior to 1955, see *National Health Programs,,* Hearings before the Senate Committee on Education and Labor on S. 1606, 79th Cong, 2d Sess, *1946, passim.* See also *America's Health, Official Report of the National Health Assembly,* Harper & Brothers, New York, 1949, *passim*; Building America's Health, *President's Commission on the Health Needs of the Nation. Government Printing Office, Washington, DC, 1952, Vol II; Campbell, RR; Campbell, WW:* "Compulsory health insurance: the economic issues." *Quarterly Journal of*

*Economics, February, 1952; Davis,* op cit.

22. *On the mounting costs of hospital care, see Hayes, JH: Factors Affecting the Costs of Hospital Care,* Vol I of *Report on Financing Hospital Care in the United States,* Blakiston Division, New York, McGraw-Hill Book Company, Inc., 1954. For the incidence of medical costs on families in 1953, see Anderson, OW: *National Family Survey of Medical Care Costs and Voluntary Health Insurance; Preliminary Report.* Chicago, Health Information Foundation, 1954. This report is partially reprinted in *Characteristics of the Low-income Population and Related Federal Programs.*

23. For an account of the various plans, see *Health Insurance Plans in the United States,* Senate Committee on Labor and Public Welfare, SR 359, 82d Cong 1st Sess, 1951, Vols. 1-3; Dickinson, FG, Falk, IS: Medical care insurance: Lessons from voluntary and compulsory plans. *American Journal of Public Health,* May 1951 (two articles); the articles by Schmidt, EP, Hall, H, McNary, WS, Hayden, CG; and Miller, JH in *Building America's Health* A Report to the President's Commission on the Health Needs of the Nation, Vol IV, *Financing a Health Program for America,* Washington, DC, Government Printing Office, 1952; *A Look at Modern Health Insurance,* US Chamber of Commerce, Washington, DC, 1954. For an account of more recent proposals see Chapters 8 and 9 below.

24. "Voluntary Insurance against Sickness: 1948-53 Estimates," *Social Security Bulletin,* December 1954, 7. The survey of the Health Information Foundation (see note 22 above) suggests that only 15% of charges incurred by families was covered by insurance in 1953.

25. For a succinct evaluation of voluntary health insurance in America, see Goldmann, F: Voluntary medical care insurance: Achievements and shortcomings. *Journal of the National Medical Association,* July 1954, 223-232.

26. For an evaluation of progress in regard to some of the more prominent serious diseases, see *Health Inquiry,* Preliminary Report of the Committee on Interstate and Foreign Commerce, Union Calendar 499, 83d Cong, 2d Sess, HR 1338, 1954.

# PART 3

# 1965: A TURNING POINT

# 5    The Social Security Amendments of 1965

Less than a year has elapsed since the Social Security Amendments of 1965 were passed, and it is already evident that this law will go down in history as the most important piece of social legislation enacted in this country since the original Social Security Act of 1935, which still has pride of place. In the health field alone, however, the 1965 law can claim to be of first importance. Despite its limitations to the aged and to certain carefully defined categories of needy or medically needy persons, its impact on every aspect of the provision of health or medical care has already been tremendous. Its implementation is making enormous demands on the time and energies and sense of public spirit of the professions concerned, on organized suppliers of health services, on hospitals and other medical institutions, and on governmental agencies.

And yet I venture to suggest that we are only at the beginning of what may well be a revolution in our methods of organizing and financing health services. After a period of digesting the measures enacted in 1965, I am convinced that we shall see further action to bring us closer to achievement of the goal so well stated by The New York Academy of Medicine˙ that "all people have the assurance of an equal opportunity to obtain a high quality of comprehensive health care." As one studies the history of social legislation one fact becomes very clear: it is that if a new policy or program is found to be good, even though initially limited in scope, there will be pressure to extend it to other groups of people or to other problem areas. And this pressure

Delivered as the keynote address of the 1966 Health Conference of the New York Academy of Medicine, *New Directions in Public Policy for Health Care*, April 21 and 22, 1966, and published under the title "Some major policy decisions facing the United States in the financing and organization of health care" in the *Bulletin of the New York Academy of Medicine*, Vol XLII, No 12 (December 1966), 1072-1088. Reprint by permission of the Academy.

will not be unduly weakened even if it emerges that a more comprehensive program costs much more than was originally thought. If people are satisfied with a program they are prepared to pay for it. In this respect and in this respect only I find myself on the same side as the American Medical Association, which has always asserted that the enactment of even a modest social insurance program would be the thin edge of the wedge of further governmental action. Needless to say, however, we differ in the emotional responses we make to this probability. The Association trembles and I rejoice.

## Some Major Policy Issues

While the 1965 legislation will surely be no end but rather a beginning, it is a very important beginning for it embodies policies that are bound to influence future developments for good or bad. We need to be very clear as to what these major policy issues are so that if change is needed it can be accomplished before it is too late or, if a choice faces us, that we be aware of the alternatives and their implications. In fact, we have many choices, for the 1965 amendments embody many different and even conflicting principles.

### Health Care as a Right or a Concession
Perhaps the most crucial of all policy issues concerns the principle on which governmentally financed health services are to be made available to people. Last year we simultaneously enacted two different principles. On the one hand, in Title 18, specified health services became available to the aged as a right through the application of the social insurance principle. On the other hand, under Title 19, various categories of needy people will be provided health care on a means test basis. Which of the two different approaches do we wish to promote in the future? Shall the social insurance approach continue to be limited to those 65 and over or should it be extended to cover some or all of those under that age? Should efforts be made to broaden the coverage of Title 19 (medical assistance on a means test basis) not only to provide federal financing for the general assistance recipients but also progressively to raise the income limits so as to include an ever larger segment of the population?

### Comprehensive Care or Item-by-Item Provisions
A second major policy decision is whether governmental financing of health services is to be made available only for specific types of health services on an item-by-item basis or is to cover all care needed by the

covered population on a comprehensive basis. Here again two different policies are embodied in the 1965 law. In Title 18 the item-by-item approach has been adopted. Only so much hospitalization or post-hospital institutional treatment will be underwritten by government. Only certain types of hospital services will be reimbursable. Ambulatory care in hospitals, extended institutional care, drugs provided outside the hospital, dental care, and many other items of normal health care are excluded. Similarly, in Title 18 B, physicians' services are to be provided and financed on an item-by-item basis. In Title 19, however, in principle, governmental financing is to be available for comprehensive health services although in the first instance the states are required to supply only five broadly defined types of care. As we plan for the future, which of the two principles do we wish to follow?

### The Respective Roles for the Federal Government and the States

So far I have spoken only of major policy issues: of the ends we wish to achieve. But important policy issues are also raised by the methods we have adopted to attain these ends. The first of these concerns the respective roles of the federal and state and local governments. Here again, we have followed two roads in the 1965 law. On the one hand we have two wholly federal programs (Hospitalization Insurance and Supplementary Medical Insurance). For although the state health authorities and private intermediaries also play a role, it is as agents of the federal government, which alone carries final responsibility for financing and policy formation. On the other hand in Medical Assistance we have what is essentially a state (or state and local) program where, although there is very substantial federal financial participation and a set of federal standards that for extensiveness surpass those of any previous grant-in-aid program, the initiative, and within quite wide limits, the nature and extent of the program rest in the hands of the states.

A major policy question for the future is thus whether to increase the role of the federal government or that of the states. And it is a decision that must take account of existing federal and state responsibilities in health areas other than those affected by the 1965 amendments, where the trend appears to be toward a growing federal responsibility for construction, research, education and, more recently, the treatment of specific diseases.

### The Role of Private Enterprise in Government Programs

A second policy issue raised by the implementing methods we have adopted concerns the role of private enterprise in what are essentially governmental programs. Here again we have started out on two paths. On the one hand, in Title 18 the legal structure provides for, although it does not require, the use of private intermediaries to perform many of the administrative functions of the programs. On the other hand, in Title 19 there is no provision for intermediaries unless the state decides to "buy into" the supplementary medical insurance for its aged needy persons. It seems likely that the use of private intermediaries in the social insurance programs was a political concession designed to overcome some of the opposition to Medicare on the part of organized medicine and the profit and nonprofit insurance companies. But what may have been politically expedient to secure enactment may or may not prove to be socially desirable once a program is established and in operation. Already some serious questions have been raised about this policy decision. As the program moves into operation it will be of the utmost importance to study experience and evaluate the wisdom of this use of private organizations in the administration of a governmental program.

The private enterprise concept is also evident in the methods adopted for the remuneration of professional personnel. Here, the policy of paying for professional services on the basis of the "reasonable charge for the service rendered" perpetuates the fee-for-service method of payment so dear to our private enterprise-oriented medical profession. As long as we conceive of the physician as a private enterpriser selling his services for the best price he can get from anyone who can afford to pay for them, the fee-for-service method of payment may make sense, though in that case one might then wonder what justification there is for governmental action to assure minimum collections and, if the doctor decides to bill the patient directly, to make possible the collection of more when the traffic will bear it. But the question that must be decided in the future is how far this concept of medicine as a private-enterprise undertaking is appropriate to a governmentally financed and operated program.

The "private enterprise" character of the market for health services has also permeated another feature of the insurance programs. The provisions for deductibles and for coinsurance, to the extent they were not inserted as political strategy to keep initial cost down, can be justified only on the assumption that the buyer too looks on health services or medical care as he looks on automobiles or any other commodity. If it is cheap he will buy or use more of it, so deductibles and coinsurance are utilized to keep demand to a minimum. But is the parallel exact? Or must we realize that to the buyer health is not like other commodities and that the money barrier of the deductible may prevent some people from seeking care when they need it, especially care of a preventive character or an early diagnosis, while coinsurance will still leave some patients with a sizable bill or the unfortunate necessity of foregoing some type of treatment or care.

### *Administration by Health or Welfare Agencies*

A third major policy issue in the implementation of the new programs concerns the allocation of administrative responsibilities among state agencies. Once again two roads have been simultaneously revealed. In Title 18 the various functions in connection with the social insurances that are delegated to the states are to be carried out by the departments of health. In Title 19 the states can designate whatever state agency they wish to administer the program although the determination of financial eligibility must be done by the welfare department. And at the federal level administrative responsibility for Title 19 is lodged in the Welfare Administration, with the Public Health Service serving only in an advisory and consultative relationship. The question of which agency shall have administrative responsibility for the enormously important Title 19 programs must not be viewed merely as a struggle for power between two governmental agencies. The decision, as I shall try to show later, has far-reaching consequences for the future development of our health services.

## The Determinants of Policy

Time does not permit the enumeration of all the many policy issues we face, and I have necessarily had to be selective. I have chosen five that seem to me to be crucial for the future development of our governmentally financed and administered health services. I am no better prepared than anyone else to forecast what answers we shall have given 25 years hence. But I am sure that in the last resort what happens will depend on the importance the people of the United States attach to certain values and objectives. Specifically, I shall try to show how the importance attached to the concept of health care as a right, to equality of access to health services, to high quality of care, to an orderly organization for the provision of health services and to economy in the use of resources devoted to health will influence our policy decisions, not only on the five major issues as I see them but also on others as well.

## The Importance Attached to Health Care as a Right

In a recent policy statement The New York Academy of Medicine says "The availability of health services, as a matter of human right should be based on health needs alone, not on a test of ability to pay." This is of course what the social insurance technique, as opposed to medical assistance, achieves, and it is of the utmost importance that we understand the implications of the two approaches. The essence of social insurance is that whatever benefits are included in the program are made available as a right, subject only to proof of insured status and the existence of the condition calling for health care. No account is taken of the economic status of the claimant at the time he is in need of care. Proof of insured status, in turn, involves the application of objective tests that are specified in the law and apply to all covered persons. They typically leave little room for argument or the exercise of official discretion in the individual case. It is this objective, non-discretionary method of determining eligibility that accounts for the great popularity of social insurance among our independent self-respecting citizens and that, incidentally, justifies prevailing terminology. For we always speak of social insurance *claimants,* whereas those whose eligibility is based on passage of a means or needs test are referred to as *applicants.* And no one likes to be an applicant.

Still less is the position of the applicant an enviable one when we look at the reality of the means test as it is typically applied by departments of welfare in the United States to applicants for public assistance. Detailed reporting of all income and other resources and of expenditure needs, verification of all statements by house visits, confirming reports from relatives, employers, landlords, and often neighbors, coupled with the exercise of wide discretion in the withholding or granting of specific items that are not included in the basic budget and, in far too many instances, the arbitrary application of additional eligibility criteria relating to the behavior of the applicant—all these explain why the means test as the door to social services is so heartily detested, not only by those who must undergo it, but also by all observers of the effect on human dignity and morale of submission to this kind of treatment.

It is true that the 1965 legislation contains a number of provisions designed to render the needs test, as applied to eligibility for medical assistance, less offensive and deterrent. Relatives' responsibility has been greatly narrowed. Only resources actually available, rather than presumably so, are to be taken into account. Arbitrary income limits that would exclude people regardless of the size of their medical bills have been ruled out. Resources must be "reasonably" evaluated.

110

Furthermore, the federal welfare administration is urging the states to simplify the needs test and the verification process. And, in theory, there would be no legal barrier to prevent a state that so desired from setting very high income limits, using income tax returns or simple affidavits for verification purposes and with predetermined eligibility wherever possible, in effect turning its Title 19 program into a full-fledged state health service, available to almost everyone. It could do this and still claim federal matching for all those whose age, family composition, or physical disabilities identified them as persons who, but for the size of their incomes, would be eligible for federally aided categorical public assistance.

I emphasize "in theory," for it is highly unlikely that this will happen on any large scale. However, if there are no further extensions of the social insurance principle to other age groups we are likely to see very extensive liberalization of medical assistance in this direction in some of our wealthier and/or more progressive states in the next few years. Realistically, however, we must expect that for the vast majority of the states the means test for health care, apart from the statutory restrictions already referred to, will be administered in a manner and a spirit that is not different from that applied to the applicant for public assistance.

This is more likely in view of the unfortunate provision in the 1965 amendments that the financial eligibility requirements must be administered by the welfare departments. One would have thought that our best chance of developing a nondeterrent, liberal, and nonoffensively administered income test for health services would have been to have lodged its administration in the hands of agencies not identified with a long tradition of deterrence, namely the health departments. After all, many of our other social programs, such as housing or educational scholarships, involve the application of an income test, but its administration is not, for that reason, lodged in the departments of welfare.

If we desire to move toward the objective of medical care as a right we shall surely push for further extension of the social insurance approach and change our administrative arrangements in medical assistance. We shall also find it necessary to reconsider our policies on deductibles and coinsurance. For if, as indicated by administration spokesmen, the two parts of Medicare will cover only between 40 and 60% of the individual's medical bill, many of the aged will discover that all that has happened is that they now must go to a welfare department to meet 60 to 40% of their bills instead of 100% as previously. They will not have been spared the necessity of contact with a means test system and they will have the added disadvantage of having to deal with two agencies.

At the same time we must never forget that social insurance is only one way of implementing the right to needed health services (see discussion in Chapter 4). It is a useful social invention that has made it possible for societies troubled about the possible effect of free payments or services on initiative and self-dependence to accept the idea of conferring rights freed from any needs-test requirement. Its contributory character supported the parallel with private insurance and made it possible to argue that people had earned their rights because they had contributed toward their benefits. But by the same token, those who had not contributed or had not made a sufficient number of contributions for whatever reason, within or beyond the individual's power to control, are denied benefits under social insurance systems. In other words, insured status as the door to rights to service inevitably excludes some people. Exclusion from benefits may under some circumstances make sense in a cash-payment program, but do we want to exclude anyone from needed health services?

Rights to services can be conferred, however, without making eligibility depend on insured status. In this country we already do this for veterans with service-connected disabilities. Some other countries, of which Great Britain is the most prominent example, have extended this right to all people who, while in Great Britain, need medical care. They treat health services, in other words, as we treat elementary and high school education. Is there any reason why health services should be less universally required than education?

Thus if we are really committed to the idea that health services should be available as a human right based on health need alone, perhaps we should raise our sights and move toward a free health service for at least some sections of the population. Children suggest themselves as the obvious target for such a service.

### The Importance Attached to Equal Access to Appropriate Health Services for All Our People

A second major determinant of future developments in the organization and financing of health services will be the importance we attach to equality of access on a geographical basis. Because of the limited scope of Title 18 in terms of persons covered, types of health service insured against, and the presence of deductibles and co-insurance, it is Title 19 that we shall find it necessary to rely on as the main instrument for ensuring that no one who needs health services is denied them. And Title 19 deals only with that part of inability to secure needed care that is due to financial inability to pay for it. It does not deal with such other obstacles as the nonavailability of personnel or facilities.

Even as a means of solving the problem of financial incapacity I fear that Title 19, despite its high potential, will result in great geographical inequalities in care. Its full implementation will involve large additional expenditures on the part of the states, which are already finding themselves under heavy pressure to finance growing educational and other state-supported services. More important is the fact that there is great variation in the per capita income of the different states. Even with the best will in the world and with an 83% federal matching, some states will be unable to raise the necessary sums. In addition, state attitudes vary greatly. Not all of them are convinced of the importance of making health services available under self-respecting conditions to everyone, especially if a large number of the beneficiaries are likely to be nonwhites or people such as unmarried mothers, who are held in social disesteem.

As a result we are likely to find wide variation from state to state in the Title 19 program (just as we did, incidentally, in the Kerr-Mills Act, of which much of Title 19 is an extension and broadening). There will be vast differences in the range and quality of services offered and in the income limits that will determine how many people benefit from the program. We may even find that some states, when they realize all the conditions they must satisfy to benefit from the Title 19 federal grants, may prefer not to participate at all and that, as 1970 approaches, the date by which states can no longer secure grants for vendor payments under the old public assistance formula, and it is compliance with Title 19 or nothing, that we shall find great political pressure to postpone the deadline.

Inequality of access to health services on a state-by-state basis may be regarded by some as the inevitable price we pay for our much vaunted federal form of government and our desire to leave maximum freedom to the states. But if growing importance comes to be attached to ensuring equality of access to high quality health care for all our people we are likely to see a much greater degree of federal involvement. Because it will be difficult to pretend that the program is really a "state" program if federal matching goes much above the already high 83%, I suspect that federal involvement will take the form not of additional federal matching but of the assumption of additional wholly federal responsibility for certain categories of people or for certain types of disease or for certain components of health services such as medical education, the construction of hospitals, of nursing

113

homes, or of health centers.

If we are to select certain categories of people as the beneficiaries of new federal programs we need to weigh our priorities carefully. So far we have selected the aged. Children, unless they are crippled or retarded or suffering specific handicaps, have been given no priority although one would have thought that a rational society would have given them the highest preference. It is true that under Title 19 all children under 21 must be covered under medical assistance if they meet the financial eligibility criteria and that a small sum is available for demonstration projects providing comprehensive health services for needy children, but as I have just indicated, these criteria and the scope of services are likely to vary greatly from state to state. The task for the years ahead is to redress the balance in favor of children, wherever they may live.

### The Importance Attached to the Objectives of High Quality Medical Care

A deep concern for high standards of service would surely have led us to lodge administrative responsibility for Title 19 clearly in the hands of health departments rather than in welfare departments (with a provision for appropriate consultation and cooperation with health agencies). At best, administration by welfare will lead to a parallel organization, the creation of an almost wholly health administrative unit within welfare departments. At worst it will create the danger of perpetuating a two-standard system: one for the means-test population and one for the rest. Even if, as it appears to be envisaged in New York, the responsibility for standard setting and control of quality is delegated to health departments, we are creating a most difficult situation in which one agency calls the tune and another pays the piper. Given the well-known proclivity of legislators at both state and federal levels to be more liberal in granting funds for functions labelled "health" than for those labelled "welfare," which typically seem to have the lowest appeal to appropriating bodies, it is unfortunate that the vast new medical assistance program was not clearly identified as a "health" rather than a "welfare" program.

I am second to none in my admiration for the welfare departments of our country which, in the majority of cases, have shown a commendable concern for the well-being of their clients and are carrying out, often with conspicuous success, an important and difficult task and one for which they receive little public recognition and much abuse. And there is much justice in the claim of the spokesmen for welfare that in the country as a whole the health departments are not as highly developed as the welfare departments, that they have taken a very narrow view of their functions and have resisted involvement in programs of direct service to people that might create for them difficult administrative relationships with the medical profession. Yet I venture to suggest that this is a short-range view, and one that disregards history. For the short run I agree that under the vigorous and imaginative leadership of the federal welfare administration and of some of our state welfare departments the new programs will get off to a quicker start and that the administrative interpretations will display more knowledge and concern for the needs of the clients than would have been the case had administration been lodged in the health departments. Yet for the long run a necessary condition for placing emphasis on quality, for bringing some order out of the present medical chaos, and for the development of policies that do not involve one set of standards for the assistance patient and another for the rest of us, is the creation of strong health departments. What the welfare spokesmen forget is their own history. Before 1935 welfare departments with experience in making cash payments and administering services con-nected therewith did not exist in many parts of the country, and those that did took a very narrow view of their responsibilities. It was the Social Security Act of 1935 which, by providing federal funds for public assistance (including its administration) coupled with the requirement that these funds be administered or supervised by a single state agency and accompanied by federal standard-setting, stimulated the development of the great welfare departments that we know today. It is sad to think that we missed the opportunity to do the same for state and local health departments in 1965.

### The Importance Attached to an Orderly Organization
### for the Provision of Health Services
An orderly organization for the provision of health services would include coverage of all health needs from prevention to rehabilitation, the elimination of gaps in service, the assurance of continuity of care, the avoidance of duplication or overlapping, and the prevalence of knowledge as to what is available and where to go to get it.

The more importance we attach to this objective, the more we shall surely move away from the item-by-item approach where separate units or types of care are identified and paid for with public funds while others are not. No word has appeared more frequently in medical literature and in health conferences in recent years than the word "fragmentation," and it has been used as a term of abuse. The item-by-item approach adopted in Title 18 can only intensify that fragmentation.

But more is needed than avoidance of intensification of fragmentation through our public programs, important as this is. Given the existence of both public and private operation of a great variety of health programs and services, a situation we shall face in this country for many years to come, there is a crying need to create a structure whereby some central health planning agency or council, on the community, state, and federal levels, is given responsibility for looking at the provision as a whole, is given authority to do something about it, and is adequately financed to do the job. Of all the innovations contained in the British National Health Service Act none in my judgment has been more far-reaching in effect than the implementation of the first sentence of Part III of the famous White Paper on Health Policy of 1944, namely: "If people are to have a right to look to a public service for all their medical needs, it must be somebody's duty to see that they do not look in vain." It has been this centralization of responsibility for looking at the structure as a whole (lodged in Britain in the Minister of Health) which, more than anything else, has stimulated critical inquiry into all aspects of the health services. It is this which has led to the many improvements which, as all students of the National Health Service in Britain know, are slowly transforming what was a 19th-century system of services into one more appropriate to the needs and scientific knowledge of the 20th century.

Concern with the nature of the over-all provision can hardly be expected of the administrators of a social insurance system, even with as dedicated and public-spirited a leadership as we fortunately have in the Social Security Administration. More especially is this so when social insurance is concerned with meeting only the costs of specific items of care. But even with more comprehensive social insurance systems the social insurance agencies have typically been concerned with structural organization and the availability of facilities and personnel only when existing structure leads to cost escalation (a subject to which I shall return) or when the lack of facilities and personnel to provide the specific services contracted for is so glaring that the program is in danger of falling into disrepute. I suspect we shall see something of this kind happening in regard to the supply of nursing homes and medical personnel as Title 18 goes into full effect.

The more we are concerned with a rational organization of health services, the more we shall question the wisdom of the use of the private intermediary, especially the profit-making insurance companies. Unless their functions are very narrowly confined to the mechanics of paying bills, and it does not look as if they will be, their existence as an integral part of the administrative structure can only complicate the task of community planning. They are not community-based or community-oriented. As fiscal agents paying on an item-by-item basis they are unlikely to be concerned with the appropriateness and adequacy of available services. At best they create yet one more agency that has to be brought into the planning process.

### The Importance Attached to Economy in the Use of Resources Devoted to Health Care

It is obvious that the implementation of the policies and programs to which we are even now committed will require the allocation of a greater proportion of our national resources to the health services. More people will be entitled to claim the services of professionals and to utilize medical institutions. The quality of the institutional care for which they are eligible will be superior to that previously received because the aged can now claim semiprivate rather than ward care and because, as a condition of participating in the program, hospitals and nursing homes will be held to higher standards. The funds devoted to the health services will also be increased because of the payment to suppliers on the basis of reasonable charges or costs. No longer will services to the indigent be paid for at submarket rates.

The costs, in the sense of the volume of resources devoted to health services, will inevitably rise. How high they go will depend in the last resort on the priority people attach to health services as opposed to the other things they could have bought with the same amount of money. And in passing I should like to disabuse those who think costs can be kept down by fixing, as a matter of policy, a maximum sum that can be spent on the health services. For, as I said earlier, if people want something badly enough they will, if necessary, give up other things to get it. But all this only emphasizes the importance of economy in the use of resources devoted to health care, and I was glad to see that The New York Academy of Medicine's policy statement emphasized "the importance of using the nation's resources in the most effective and economical manner consistent with the enhancement of individual dignity and high standards of care."

But if we are really concerned about economizing resources, would we have adopted what is essentially a major-medical type of insurance in Title 18B? All experience has shown that this method of reimbursement tends to escalate costs by making it easier for suppliers to raise prices or to provide unnecessary services. Would we have fragmented our governmentally financed services, thereby running the risk that, for instance, people may find it necessary to utilize costly hospitals because there is no provision for reimbursing hospital-based

117

ambulatory care? Would we have envisaged the involvement of private intermediaries in control of utilization? Even now the effectiveness of utilization committees run by the professionals concerned is very uneven. How much more concern for the public interest in economy of use can we expect when assistance to hospitals and related agencies "in the application of safeguards against unnecessary utilization of services" is placed in the hands of competitive profit-making concerns whose orientation will surely be primarily toward what makes life easy for their clients and attractive to themselves as administrators? A concern for economy in the use of resources would surely have led us to make provision for more effective representation of the public interest on the many committees that are setting policy in the application of the "reasonable cost" provisions. It might have led us to make arrangements for the separate organization of consumers of the health services who are also taxpayers, to counter the pressures of organized medicine and the insurance companies on the federal agency. The short time elapsing between passage of the act and its coming into effect means that many major policy decisions and interpretations must be made in a hurry and, inevitably under such circumstances, existing organizations exert what in retrospect may well come to be seen as an undue influence. No aspect of our new programs is in more need of study and reconsideration than the provision made for proper representation of the public interest, for publicity, and for accountability.

Waste, in the sense of more resources being devoted to a particular service than is really necessary, occurs not only when patients are kept in costly facilities because equally appropriate but less costly methods of caring for them are not available or not reimbursable, or when suppliers, through the exercise of monopoly power, are able to charge an excessive price for their services. It also occurs when procedures that could be performed by less highly trained personnel under professional supervision are carried out by expensively trained professionals. It occurs when unnecessary tests or procedures are applied. It occurs when too many hospitals are built in a community or when there are too many acute general beds or hospital laboratories or when, for prestige considerations, individual hospitals create specialist departments, as for brain surgery or cobalt treatments, which in total are far in excess of the total community need.

A concern for economy in these respects will lead ultimately, I am convinced, to a reconsideration of the status and independence of the voluntary hospital. Given the large proportion that hospital costs form of the medical bill, given the many possibilities of reducing costs (as itemized, for instance, by the Folsom Report in New York) of which

118

the hospitals could have, but have not, taken advantage, given the importance of assuring a uniform accounting system to permit effective interhospital cost comparisons and given finally the crucial importance of the hospital in the total organization of health services, we cannot much longer permit the voluntary hospital to operate as a purely private concern, answerable only to its own governing board. The recent so-called Folsom Law, which introduces a measure of public control over hospital expansion and operation, is a significant straw in the wind. And I wish to add that what I have said about the essentially "public-interest" character of the voluntary hospitals applies equally to "private" health insurance, both profit and nonprofit. All of them are, in fact, public social utilities.

In our concern about economy in the use of resources devoted to health care we must, however, never forget that in the broader sense waste also occurs when we continue to treat as exclusively medical problems conditions that might be prevented by appropriate policy and program changes in other areas, such as housing, or the reduction of poverty, or the improvement of education.

## The Agenda for the Future

I have tried to suggest to you that the problem of how we organize and finance medical care has by no means been answered by the Social Security Amendments of 1965, important as they are. Even within the limited areas with which the act is concerned, essentially the aged, the indigent, and the medically indigent, a number of highly questionable and sometimes conflicting policies have been adopted. But it has started us on a road from which there can be no returning. Governmental involvement in the financing and organization of our health services is here to stay and there is every indication that it will increase. Resolution of the policy issues at stake provides an agenda that will make the greatest demands on our ingenuity and our resourcefulness for the rest of this century. It will also make great demands on our courage and our sense of public responsibility. Above all, it will be a crucial test of the strength of our conviction that all people should have the assurance of an equal opportunity to obtain a high quality of comprehensive health care under self-respecting conditions.

# 6 Social Policy and the Health Services: The Choices Ahead

There appears to be universal agreement that the passage of the Social Security Amendments of 1965 opened a new era for the health services. On all sides one meets the expectation that nothing will ever be the same again. And yet at first sight it is not obvious why this should be so. For at least in comparison with the social policies of other countries, what was enacted by the 1965 amendments was modest indeed. Our adoption in Title 18A of the principle of compulsory social insurance was extremely timid. We limit it to paying for hospital and certain types of hospital-related care, and indeed only to some types of care received in hospitals. And the benefits are restricted to people 65 and over. This must seem a very conservative step to the over 50 countries which have, in some cases for generations, used compulsory health insurance as the basic method for meeting the costs of health and medical care with no age restriction on the beneficiaries.[1] Even in the United States the use of social insurance for health care is not entirely new. We have utilized for half a century a primitive form of social insurance, namely workmen's compensation, to pay for the costs of medical care received by those suffering from occupationally connected injuries or illnesses.

The use in Title 18B of a different method of meeting the costs of physician and certain other services, different in that coverage is voluntary rather than compulsory and in that people have to continue to pay premiums instead of benefiting from fully paid-up insurance at age 65, while the benefits take the form of indemnification or

Delivered as the Sixth Annual Bronfman Lecture at the Ninety-fourth Annual Meeting of the American Public Health Association and reprinted by permission from the *American Journal of Public Health,* Vol LVII, No 2, February 1967, 199-212.

reimbursement rather than service, involves no major departure from our well-established systems of private insurance.

Even the potentially more radical Title 19 which opens the door to an extension of free health services to those higher up the income scale than the public assistance recipients must seem a very tiny step toward universal access to needed health services to countries such as Great Britain, which operate a comprehensive national health service available to everyone regardless of income. In any case, Title 19 is primarily an extension to more people of a policy we had already adopted in the Kerr-Mills Act of 1960.

Yet I believe the general view that things have changed is justified. The 1965 amendments are the culminating step of a change process that has been with us for some time, and the tempo of which has greatly accelerated in recent years. Starting with the Hill-Burton Act in 1946, we have witnessed a long series of acts providing for federal aid for health research, for mental health, for community health facilities, for medical and nursing education, for training other types of health personnel, and for the health care of the medically indigent aged.[2] Historically viewed, therefore, the 1965 amendments are but one more step in this cumulative process. There are, however, three facts that justify our attaching a special importance to them. To begin with, for the first time a public medical care program has been enacted which brings people of all social classes within its scope. Except for veterans and workers covered by workmen's compensation, governmental action to help people meet their medical bills has hitherto been limited to people who are found to be poor or indigent. This inclusion of middle-class people in a publicly operated program has important consequences. For it is the unfortunate and shameful truth that by and large we have been little concerned about the quality and adequacy of the medical care received by those we classify as "poor" or "indigent." Once middle-class people are involved, however, we become more sensitive about quality of service. Means-test medicine is apparently not good enough for them. Quality standards are embodied in the legislation and the scope of government action becomes broader than the mere removal of a financial barrier.

Second, the very magnitude of the new programs places them in a different category from previous legislation. As a federal program Title 18 is in effect in all parts of the country, the people covered run into millions, and the dollar costs into billions. More people who, remember, are voters, will have a stake in how the program operates. Perhaps even more significantly for the long run, the administrators of public programs have to be accountable to the public and accountability means visibility. From now on we shall have much more adequate and precise information about the availability, adequacy, and costs of our health services in the nation as a whole and in its various subdivisions. The alibi of ignorance will be ever harder to maintain and the pressure for reform will be intensified.

Third, the 1965 amendments were passed in the face of the active and highly publicized opposition of organized medicine. By the very violence and duration of its opposition to compulsory health insurance the American Medical Association has unfortunately created the impression that it was challenging the right of the people to use their government to achieve objectives to which they attached importance. Inevitably, therefore, passage of the legislation is viewed as a "victory," symbolizing and legitimating once and for all the fact that there is indeed a public interest in health and that the opinions of professional groups cannot prevail when in conflict with that interest. Never again will the medical profession be able to assert, as it did in 1946 when testifying on the National Health Program Bill, that doctors and only doctors were "in a position to pass upon the medical side of it, as to the determination of medical care and how to obtain it, and the effect upon medical care of the system."[3] Already this assertion has an archaic sound.

## The Main Issues

Now that it is established that the functioning of our health services is a legitimate concern of social policy and that public action will be invoked when necessary, it is imperative that we clarify the ends of policy, assess the efficacy of available ways of obtaining them, and reformulate the role of the professional and other groups who must play a part in the enterprise. The overall goal is not difficult to define. The New York Academy of Medicine summarized it for us when, in a recent policy statement, they asserted that all people should have the assurance of an equal opportunity to obtain a high quality of comprehensive health care and that the availability of services should be based on health needs alone and not on ability to pay.[4] In moving toward that goal there would seem to be three important choices facing the nation.[5] First, shall the financial barrier to receipt of health services be lowered for more people and, if so, how? Second, shall social policy be concerned solely with removing the financial barrier? Third, is the primary concern of social policy with health services or with health?

# Should the Financial Barrier Be Removed
# or Lowered for More People and, If So, How?

The main thrust and the main novelty of the 1965 legislation has been the deliberate use of social policy to remove or lower the financial barrier to access to health services. As we all know, this has been achieved by the use of compulsory, and voluntary federally subsidized, insurance for the benefit of people 65 and over, and by increasing the numbers who can secure publicly financed medical services through a liberalization of the concept of indigency. It seems inevitable in the years ahead that insistent questions will be raised as to the desirability of limiting access to these programs to the presently covered groups. Specifically, we shall surely see (indeed we are already seeing) demands for the extension of social insurance to benefit groups other than the aged, and efforts within the states to broaden the coverage of Title 19 by progressive increases in the income limits.

### The Limits of Voluntary Private Insurance

How far these extensions will go will depend mainly on the degree to which existing private arrangements for the financing of health services prove able to remove or sufficiently moderate the financial barrier for those not now benefiting from Titles 18 and 19. Great hopes are being placed on the ability of private insurance, freed as it now is from the impossible burden of trying to solve the problem of the health costs of the aged, to expand its coverage of both population groups and types of service. Yet despite the levels of affluence of this country which suggest that the potential is great, it seems highly unlikely that private insurance coverage can be extended sufficiently widely and rapidly to ward off demands for further extensions of governmental programs. The percentage of the population with coverage declines sharply as income falls.[6] Much of the rapid extension of coverage of the past has taken the form of health fringe benefits as part of the collective bargaining system. The better-off and the organized workers are the groups that have been easy to reach. But what of the employees of small firms, the domestic servants, and agricultural workers? What of the increasing numbers of older but not yet aged workers, many suffering from a variety of disabilities that limit their capacity to take employment, or the families that have lost their breadwinner through death? Nor will it be easy to deny the claims of the increasing numbers of older people who have exercised their socially accorded right to retire at age 62 and who will surely question the sacredness of age 65, more especially as the pre-65 retiree will necessarily be drawing a benefit that is lower than that of the worker who retired at age 65?

It seems inevitable that there will be sizable groups for whom protection through private insurance is an unrealistic hope. Even more uncertain is the ability of private insurance to offer even approximately complete protection for the population groups who are insured. Deductibles, coinsurance, indemnity payments that fail to reflect rising costs of service, and exclusion of important components of medical care help to explain why by 1964 private insurance met only 33% of all consumer expenditures on medical care.[7] Even if the industry is able to maintain rates of increase in cost coverage characteristic of the last three years (actually since 1961 the rate has slightly slowed down) it will be 20 years before more than half of consumer expenditures will be reimbursed.

### Governmental Methods of Removing the Financial Barrier

If dissatisfaction with the achievements and distrust of the potential of private insurance should lead to demands for the extension of governmental programs to groups not now covered, a choice will have to be made as to which type of program is to be expanded. We have available three major technics for overcoming the financial barrier. People may be given access to health services because they are judged by the community to have incomes and resources too small to enable them to meet their medical bills (i.e., they become eligible on passage of a needs test), or because they have in the past paid taxes (euphemistically called contributions) as members of a social insurance system (i.e., eligibility rests on the concept of insured status), or because they are members of a population group for whose health status the community feels a particular concern. The last group it should be noted may be as small as presidents, and important public figures, as sizable as veterans with service-connected disabilities, or nursing mothers and their babies, or as large as the entire population.

There is an important difference between the needs-test eligibility criterion and the other two. The latter give access to health services on the basis of legally specified, nondiscretionary criteria. The beneficiaries are claimants and not applicants and are not subjected to the humiliating procedures typical of most means-test administration in the past. The absence of a test of income in systems of social insurance or free health services has another important consequence. As I have already indicated, the groups eligible are sizable and, economically, much more representative of the entire population—they are not composed solely of "the poor or indigent" and they have a significant middle-class component. This constitutes an important safeguard against the development of two systems of medical care: one for the

125

population covered by the public program and one for everyone else.

It is, of course, not inevitable that publicly financed medical care for the needy should be of inferior quality. Indeed one of the choices we face today is whether or not to take advantage of the new funds and resources available under Title 19 to improve the quality of services instead of just giving more of the same old unsatisfactory service to more people. There are encouraging signs that in many of our communities today a new wind is blowing and efforts are indeed being made to use the funds and the powers given by Title 19 to improve the quality of service.

### Disadvantages of Income or Means Tests

Assuming that it would be possible to avoid the unfortunate perpetuation of two systems of health services, one for the needy or indigent and one for the insured or nonneedy—and it is a big assumption—the question may perhaps be asked whether there is anything inherently wrong in using an income test as the instrument for overcoming the financial barrier. After all, we use income tests to determine who shall have access to certain other social benefits such as educational scholarships or fellowships or subsidized housing as well as to determine who shall contribute toward the costs of running the government, and no one seems to feel it is degrading to fill out an application form for scholarship aid or an income tax return. Thus some would argue that given the prevailing American social philosophy regarding individual responsibility, while society is prepared to ensure that no one shall be denied needed health services because of inability to pay for them, there is no necessity to provide free or subsidized services for people who have adequate financial resources of their own. They would, therefore, hold that some kind of an economic test of eligibility is desirable. But adoption of this approach means that society will then have to come to grips with a major social policy question: Where is the line to be drawn?

Already this issue has come to the fore in the implementation of Title 19 and the anguished reaction of Congress to the relatively liberal plans of New York and some other states indicates how much difference of opinion there is in the country as to the income level which is too low to enable people to pay for the medical care they need.

In any case, we must never forget that, contrary to prevailing beliefs, the purpose of eligibility conditions is to keep people out rather than to let them in. But we do not want to exclude anyone from needed medical care. Hence, whatever the form of income test adopted, it must not be of a character that deters people from using health services when they need them. From this point of view one can only regret that the Congress so deliberately specified in Title 19 that the test of financial eligibility must be administered by welfare departments. Although some welfare administrations are endeavoring to make the test nondeterrent by using affidavits in place of detailed investigation and verification, by simplifying and formalizing the information called for and by predetermination of eligibility wherever possible, it is doubtful whether most welfare agencies can so far break with their past traditions as to operate a truly nondeterrent financial test of eligibility for health services.

Given the improbability that our poorer and our meaner states will provide first-class health services for those whose access to them is determined on the basis of need, given the unlikelihood that the test will be everywhere administered in a nondeterrent manner, and in view of the violent differences of opinion that are likely to arise as to where, in a federally aided system, the income limit should be set, I suspect that the use of an income test will not prove to be the answer to our problem. If we really wish to ensure that availability of health services should be based on health needs alone and not on the individual's ability to pay for them, we shall have to resort to one or other of the nonneeds-test technics for overcoming the financial barrier, namely, to social insurance or to free health services for specified segments of the population. For it is one of the advantages of social insurance that it enables us to evade the awkward question of the exact income level which should entitle people to free or subsidized health care. But since even social insurance excludes some people (notably, in most systems, those who are not employed), we may also find ourselves moving toward a free health service for some of our more vulnerable but strategically important groups such as children.[8]

This may not be so revolutionary as it sounds. The medical profession and the insurance companies must have had a severe shock in recent months as they have begun to see how dangerous Title 19 is from their point of view. As many of us warned them at the time, the Kerr-Mills approach which they saw as a safe alternative to social insurance had the potential in a liberal state of becoming a universally available free health service. They may yet come to regard a free health service for children as a lesser evil than the possibility of extending free services to an ever larger proportion of the entire population by a continuous raising of the income limits under Title 19.

# Shall Social Policy Be Concerned
## Solely with Removing the Financial
## Barrier?

This is perhaps the most important of all the choices we face. The stimulus to enactment of Titles 18 and 19 was a concern about the burden of medical care costs. Both the Congress and the Administration have narrowly defined the objectives of the new programs, especially of Title 18. In the words of Commissioner Ball, "The main purpose of the legislation, of course, is to help older people meet the cost of the medical care they receive. The program does not itself provide care. . . . It is our direct concern . . . to help people meet their bills, not to make changes in the way medical care is given."[9]

Consistently with this objective the new programs have started out on a pattern that interferes as little as possible with existing structural and administrative arrangements, methods of operation and remuneration, and professional mores and relationships. So far as possible every agency, every purveyor of service, every health institution is to be enabled to go about his or its business as before. Indeed, a cynic might be tempted to assert that the main beneficiaries of the new legislation will be those involved in the provision of health services. Hospitals will be paid their full reasonable costs for care given to the aged and indigent, doctors will be more sure of collecting full payment of their reasonable charges and left free to collect whatever unreasonable charges they can induce their aged patients to pay, and they can continue to insist on the fee-for-service principle. Insurance companies have been relieved of a burden and have been given a new claim on the loyalty of their customers in their capacity as helpful administrators of a large reimbursement program.

In fact, the new legislation does have some impact on "the way medical care is given." Despite the brave words of the first section of Title 18 which, you will recall, states "Nothing in this title shall be construed to authorize any federal officer or employee to exercise any supervision or control over the practice of, or the manner in which medical services are provided . . . or to exercise any supervision or control over the administration of any such institution, agency, or person," there are some controls and some supervision even now. Ironically the most serious interference with the way medical care is given was inserted at the request of organized medicine itself, which may yet live to regret the precedent it has set. I refer, of course, to the removal from Title 18A to Title 18B of in-hospital professional services. Some measure of quality control exists through the conditions laid down for institutional participation in Title 18. A limited degree of control over hospital operation is found in the requirement for utilization committees. The necessity to set national criteria for the determination of "reasonable costs and reasonable charges" theoretically makes possible some measure of social control over methods and levels of remuneration, although the composition of the advisory bodies involved, with their minuscule provisions for representation of the public interest and their overwhelmingly heavy medical and insurance membership necessarily tempers one's hopes.

### The Pressure of Costs

These controls are minimal and no more than would be necessary in any financial underwriting arrangement. The insurer, in this case the government, has contracted to meet the costs of certain kinds and levels of service and has to make sure that its customers get what they have been promised in return for their premiums. Because the program is financed on an insurance basis any rise in costs will have to be reflected in rising premiums. Because taxpayers are notoriously resistant to increased taxes even when they are called insurance contributions, government will of necessity be greatly concerned with practices or administrative arrangements that lead to rising costs. Hence, if the costs of the programs prove to be greater than originally anticipated we are likely to see more controls. If physicians' fees show a significant upward trend that coincides suspiciously with the inauguration of Medicare it will not be surprising if such a development becomes a matter of public concern and action. Questions might even be asked whether some system of payment other than fee-for-service might not result in lower costs. If hospital costs continue their spectacular rise it will be no surprise if government begins to take a hard look at the way hospitals are run with a view to reducing costs. Such developments are the more likely in that for the first time we have a national program, which greatly enlarges the possibility of making comparisons of performance on a more uniform basis. And, as I have already indicated, what is happening will be known and reported on. There will be greater visibility.

This concern with cost is unlikely to be restricted to the public programs. National expenditures for health services are large and continuously rising. In 1964 they amounted to $36.8 billions or 5.8% of GNP. In 1950, only 14 years earlier, they were only $12.9 billions or 4.5% of the then GNP. Per capita, the rise has been spectacular, from $84.50 in 1950 to $191.30 in 1964, an increase that, even when allowance is made for the rising price levels, is over 75%[10]; and there is universal agreement that further increases must be expected.

Part of the rise in national expenditures on health is, of course, due to the fact that we are demanding more of our health services and that the scientific progress of recent years has provided new procedures and methods of treatment that involve additional expense. It is also true that we are a rich nation, growing richer all the time, so that to some degree we can indeed afford to spend more on our health services as on everything else; but even rich nations have to face up to the fact that at any given time and level of national income the more they spend for one type of goods or service the less they can spend on all other possible objects of expenditure. It thus becomes of the greatest importance to assure that whatever level of service is desired shall be rendered at minimum cost in the sense of not making a greater demand than is absolutely necessary on resources which might be available for other purposes.

As the total burden of health costs increases, we may well expect demands from the public that the suppliers of health services demonstrate that they are indeed producing at minimum cost. This is already happening in the hospital insurance field where state regulatory bodies are no longer prepared to accept the insurer's argument that premiums must be increased because hospital costs have risen. They are asking with growing frequency, "Are these cost increases really necessary? Is it not possible by organizational or administrative changes to make economies without lowering quality?" In view of the sizable demand that hospitals make on our national resources we must expect more questioning of the necessity for additional hospitals, more pressure for the utilization of available beds, more challenging of the necessity for under-utilized specialized equipment, and more attention to regional planning as a way of securing economies and, if necessary, there will be public action to bring about desired changes.

When the public is told that the country needs to train 50% more physicians annually if its 1959 physician-population ratio is to be maintained by 1975, and begins to count the cost of producing them, it is inevitable that people will want to know whether we are making the best use of the physicians we now have by using them only for tasks which call for so costly a training. They may even ask whether the training need be so long and costly. We can expect increasingly insistent demands to exploit the possibility of using auxiliary personnel whose training involves a lower investment.[11]

Thus we may well expect more, rather than less, involvement of government with the way medical care is given. But note that the spur to action could remain merely a concern about cost. Even if, in the years ahead, the American people were to decide that they wished to extend the benefits of one or both parts of Title 18 to ever larger groups of the population by progressively lowering the age limit, the objectives of social policy could still remain restricted to removing the financial barrier. Even if all states were to exploit Title 19 to the full by progressively raising the income limits and including an ever broader spectrum of services, the undertaking could still be conceived of as merely a financial commitment. In both cases government's involvement with the way medical care is organized, administered, and delivered would still be restricted to those features which affect costs.

## The Pressure of Service Needs

Are the objectives of social policy to remain thus limited? I suggest that our answer to this question cannot be "yes." We all know that even if everyone could afford to pay all his medical bills or could have them paid for him, removal of the financial barrier would not automatically assure good medical care or, more importantly, a high standard of health for all.

It is not necessary to particularize the many other obstacles to the general availability of high quality and appropriate health services. The impressive body of evidence that has accumulated in recent years in commission reports, in conferences of health professionals, in articles in professional journals and in governmental publications has familiarized us all with the major weaknesses.[1][2] We are aware of the increasingly serious personnel shortages and of the inadequacies of much of our institutional provision. We know about the great geographical inequalities not only among states but within states in the availability of both personnel and facilities. The lag between new knowledge and its application is a painfully familiar theme at almost all health conferences and symposia. The deficiencies of our delivery system are notorious. The provision of health services has evolved along a series of tracks that often do not meet and are certainly not coordinated. We still retain the curious distinction between the preventive and the diagnostic and curative services and between them and the rehabilitative. We still have largely parallel systems for the treatment of physical and mental illness. We make a sharp distinction between services for the vertical (or ambulatory) patient and those for the horizontal (or hospitalized) patient, regardless of the fact that at different times the same patient may be both. We develop services on the basis of disease entities so that the care an individual gets may depend on whether he has the "right" kind of disease. We make distinctions between people for the purpose of the delivery of services that have no logical basis: special provision for public well-baby clinics but not for babies who are sick. We provide school health services to identify the health needs of school children but fail to follow through to see that deficiencies are corrected. We glorify the principle of free choice of physician, but fail to recognize that the choice that is given is primarily the selection of the door through which one gains access to a range of needed services. Thereafter, there is little free choice. If the general practitioner is incompetent or is professionally obsolete, or if he is barred from a hospital connection for reasons other than lack of appropriate qualifications, his patients are unlikely to find that free choice of physician is any guarantee of good medical care.

It is not surprising that the word "fragmentation" appears with such depressing frequency in all the recent literature or that the objective of "comprehensive care" seems to be Item I on the agenda of every proposal for reform. But if these deficiencies and weaknesses, these nonfinancial obstacles to receipt of high quality health care, are to be corrected, social policy must of necessity be concerned with the way medical care is given. There seems to be little doubt that social policy will come to grips with the problem of securing an adequate total supply of essential facilities and health personnel of all kinds. For here the major choice facing the nation is how much money it is willing to pay to achieve the objective, and all experience suggests that if people want something badly enough they will, if necessary, give up other things to get it.

The decision as to how much money to spend is one that is much easier to make than those to be faced if something is to be done to correct the geographical unevenness in the availability of facilities and personnel, or to improve our delivery systems, or to supply services at minimum cost. Solutions to these problems, whether brought about by voluntary action on the part of the professions or institutions involved or by governmental action, inevitably touch raw nerves. Professional interests that include, but go far beyond, the purely economic are threatened. Long established methods of operation and well-recognized roles may have to change. Comfortable bureaucratic habits and practices may have to be abandoned or at least be severely modified. Local political loyalties may have to be subordinated to the necessity of adopting wider and more rational areas such as regions, as the basis for planning and operation.

## Is the Primary Concern of Social Policy with Health Services or with Health?

Much of the ferment now under way or foreseeable focuses upon health services as such. We are all eager to improve their adequacy, their

132

availability and their quality, and this is not surprising. For all professions appear to suffer from what I once called "professional myopia." We tend to assume that the obvious solution to the human problems with which we deal is the provision of more and better services of the kind we have been trained to render.

Yet it is well known that the health of a people, while obviously affected by the nature of its health services and the presence or absence of contaminations in its physical environment, is also greatly influenced by other factors of a social character. Poor housing, inadequate nutrition, unwanted pregnancies, inability to secure employment, limited education, especially as it relates to elementary knowledge of the functioning of the body and mind, exclusion from participation in the ongoing life of the community, all these have a direct impact on physical or mental health and often on both.

If it is health that we are concerned with then the scope of our social policy for health must be expanded to encompass these social areas as well. It makes no sense to develop costly mental health services to undo the harm that could have been avoided if people had not been compelled to exist on inadequate incomes or forced to try to cope with essentially uncopable problems.

I must confess that those of us whose professional and civic interests involve us in so-called welfare activities, in efforts to secure sound and adequate programs in the fields of social insurance, public assistance, antipoverty legislation, education, or housing and urban renewal for instance, often have occasion to wish that we could count on more active support and cooperation from our colleagues in the health professions. For surely in this area the health professional, the economist, the sociologist, or the social worker whose professional competence lies in the area of social legislation, have a common interest—the improvement of health.

## The Challenge to the Health Professions

The answer to my three central questions will, of course, ultimately be made by the American people themselves. I believe they will insist upon change in all three areas. We can expect a demand for the further lowering of the financial barriers and for a removal of the more important nonfinancial obstacles to the receipt of medical care, for a rationalization of our present chaotic system for the delivery of health services and for improvements in the social environment that will have a favorable impact on health. The only uncertainty concerns how these changes are to be brought about and where the leadership is to come from.

Some of the needed changes can undoubtedly be accomplished by action within the private sector. Some can only be carried through by government, while in other cases public action may have to be invoked because the professions and the private health institutions fail to act when they could have done so. It is clear, too, that effective implementation of these changes will require the cooperation of many disciplines: economists, political scientists, administration experts, sociologists, and the like, as well as health professionals.

Whatever form is assumed in the future by our institutional arrangements for the financing, organization, and administration of health services, our own past experience and that of other countries has shown that the extent to which the objective of high quality comprehensive health care is attained depends in large measure on the role which the health professions themselves decide to play. Whether the final form of organization and financing be some combination of public and private action, as seems most likely, and whether public action takes the form of a broadened health insurance system, a liberalized income-tested program or a free health service for larger or smaller groups of the population, the outcome will be influenced by the nature of the participation of the professions involved. The choice they face is whether to limit their role to the protection of professional interests, narrowly conceived, or to subordinate these interests to the public interest by active participation in the process of developing adequate, universally available, economically operated, and high quality health services.

There are three groups within the health services whose decisions will be of crucial importance. The first is the medical profession itself, whose members do indeed have it within their power to withhold from the nation the expert guidance and professional help they could give by constructive participation, at every stage, in the planning and development of health policies and programs. The events of 1965 have already shown the unfortunate consequences of the withdrawn, narrow professional attitude. Medical men know what makes for good medical care and high quality and appropriate health services. In view of the importance attached in leading medical circles to the concept of "comprehensive care" I cannot believe that if the medical profession had been sharing constructively in the planning of both parts of Title 18, we would have adopted a system that treats health care as a commodity to be bought in a supermarket, item by item, with a built-in encouragement to the consumer to buy mainly those services for which the cost will be reimbursed. With all the lip service that is given to the primacy of prevention, had the medical profession been active at the planning stage the act would surely not have excluded periodic health examinations, screenings, immunizations, and eye examinations from the list of reimbursable items. Given all that is known about the limitations of solo practice, would not a law that reflected the forward thinking of the medical profession have embodied inducements to encourage group practice?

We must not underestimate the magnitude of the demand made on the medical profession in asking for their full cooperation in the exciting and challenging task of shaping and applying social policies directed toward excellence in our health services. For the agonizing decision to place public interests ahead of narrow professional interests has many consequences. It means that many members of the profession will have to give time to matters other than the treatment of patients or the conduct of research. Some of its leaders will have to devote time to that most repulsive and time-consuming of all occupations, serving on committees, committees concerned with the restructuring of our delivery systems, or the formulation of standards for practice or with negotiations on behalf of their colleagues about the forms and amounts of remuneration. It means fully accepting the responsibilities that flow from the claim that the profession should be the sole judge of what is or is not good professional practice. Some members of the profession will have to sit in judgment on others, whether it be in the functioning of utilization committees or testing qualifications for practice or, if certain systems of remuneration should be adopted, discriminating among colleagues on the basis of relative competence.

Placing the public interest ahead of narrow professional interests means also that as the key profession involved in the rendering of service, physicians must be prepared to pay more attention to the importance of economy. It means a willingness to abandon the performance of procedures and tasks that do not call for high levels of expertise and which could be performed effectively by less highly trained professional or auxiliary workers, alone or under medical supervision. It involves removal of some of the mystique of medicine by more vigorous support of efforts, starting in our schools, to disseminate to the population as a whole a better knowledge of the functioning of the body and the mind and of some of the more elementary principles of medical care; and it calls for a willingness to reassess the character of medical education itself.[13]

Admittedly this is to ask much of the medical profession. Yet, is it really more than to ask them that they should behave as true professionals? For the justification of the special privileges that society grants to a profession is its claim to place service to the community ahead of pecuniary or other personal advantage. The public image of the medical profession is unfortunately badly tarnished today.[14] Constructive participation in the new social policies might yet restore its old splendor.

The second major group faced with difficult choices consists of those concerned with the policies and administration of our hospitals and especially the voluntary general hospitals. Essentially their choice is whether to conceive of the hospital's role as being that of serving as the community medical center responsible for comprehensive health services, or continuing to be an institution concerned mainly with episodic care and serving primarily the interests of the medical profession as vehicles for teaching and as expensively equipped workshops for practitioners.

The change of role will not be easy. It will involve de-emphasizing inpatient care and, in Dr. Falk's words "upgrading ambulatory care as an equal interest rather than as an unavoidable affliction."[15] It implies also a continuing concern with what happens to the patient after he leaves the hospital, and thus an active concern with the availability and appropriateness of community health services.

But more than this is involved. Now that the health services have become a matter of social policy the voluntary hospitals must come to terms with the fact that there is indeed a public interest in what they do or do not do. This interest stems not merely from the fact that henceforth an increasing proportion of their income will come from public funds and not only because they make heavy demands on the nation's economic resources. It arises even more importantly from their strategic position in the total structure of health services. Functionally considered, they are indeed quasi-public bodies and no longer purely "private" or "voluntary." As such they can no longer be answerable for performance only to their boards of governors or to the hospital administrator or to the dominant professional groups: they are answerable to the public. Nor can their governing bodies consist only of our richer or more prominent citizens. They must reflect, because they serve, all classes of health consumers in the community.

The third group to whom the present situation presents a challenge, but also a great opportunity, consists of our public health departments and their staffs. As health becomes increasingly a matter of public concern and the subject of social policy, there will be an ever more intense need for some public agency that not only administers some of our public health programs but is also concerned with the totality of the health of our communities. I do not see how it will be possible to achieve all that is hoped for unless we can develop in all our localities and states strong and active health departments.

Dr. Luther Terry reminded us, in his Bronfman Lecture, that "the health officer and the health department remain the only agents which the body politic has been willing to pay to be concerned with the health of the public as a whole."[16]

Carrying out this mandate will however necessitate adoption of a broader view of the functions of a health department than generally appears to prevail. It will mean, as Dr. Trussell so cogently argued in his Bronfman Lecture,[17] becoming concerned with the quality of the medical care and health services available to the community. It involves a preparedness to serve as the health watchdog of the community, letting the public know what it is getting for the money it spends on its governmental and private health programs. It is no credit to our health departments or to health professionals in general that it was newspaper reporters and politicians who exposed the shameful state of the municipal hospitals in the richest city in the country. It means taking up a position, in the interests of good health care, on proposals that might prejudice the sound development of the health services. It was unfortunate, for example, that when Title 19 was being drafted, the public health departments of the country were not mobilized to insist that the expanded program be conceived of as a health and not a welfare measure and as such should be made the responsibility of departments of health. It means adopting a broader view of the concept of prevention, not limiting it to physical environmental health in the traditional sense but undertaking also investigations of the impact of social factors, for example, of low incomes or poor housing on health, and bringing the findings forcibly to the attention of the public.

This will not be easy. Operation of public medical programs, especially if they are income-tested, will indeed mean undertaking administrative tasks that traditionally have been held in low esteem when done by welfare departments. Administrative responsibility for the economical operation and high quality of a publicly financed program will create new and inevitably less cozy relationships with medical practitioners. Carrying out the mandate to be concerned with the health of the public as a whole means reaching out to the community and involving its members through advisory committees and in other ways in both evaluation and pressure for change. The broadened function will inevitably involve the health departments in controversy and they will need the support of an informed and interested public. These are big risks, yet the stakes are so high that I cannot believe the public health profession will turn its back on this great opportunity.

The new element with which we all have to come to terms and which was symbolized by the 1965 legislation is that the question of the health of the people has now been *elevated* to the realm of conscious social policy. This means that change will come and the only question is how and under what leadership. It is evident that people are intensely concerned about health and it is one of the glorious traditions of this country, more obvious perhaps to those who observe us than to ourselves, that if the American people are convinced that something is desirable and ought to be done they will find ways of doing it.

## Notes

1. *Social Security Programs Throughout the World, 1964.* Social Security Administration, US Department of Health, Education and Welfare. Washington, DC: GP Office, 1964; Hogarth J: *The Payment of the General Practitioner.* New York, Pergamon Press, 1963 (contains a useful brief description of the major European social insurance programs).

2. The tempo of legislative activity has sharply increased since 1960. Among the more important enactments (several of which have been extended or continued by subsequent amendments) are: Community Health Services and Facilities Act, 1961; Vaccination Assistance Act, 1965; Migrant's Health Act, 1962; The Community Mental Health Centers Act, 1963; the Maternal and Child Health and Mental Retardation Planning Amendments, 1963; The Mental Retardation Facilities Construction Act, 1963; Health Professions Educational Assistance Act, 1963; Clean Air Act, 1963; Hospital and Medical Facilities Amendment of 1964; Nurse Training Act, 1954; Graduate Public Health Training Amendments, 1964; Health Research Facilities Amendments, 1965; Drug Abuse Control Amendments, 1965; Heart Disease, Cancer, and Stroke Amendments, 1965; Medical Library Assistance Act, 1965; Vocational Rehabilitation Act Amendments of 1965; Comprehensive Health Planning and Public Health Service Amendments, 1966; Allied Health Professions Personnel Training Act, 1966. In addition, the Social Security Amendments of 1960 enacted the Kerr-Mills, Medical Assistance for the Aged programs, while National Institutes were established for General Medical Services (1962), and Child Health and Human Development (1964). Brief accounts of the provisions of these laws are given in *Health, Education, and Welfare Indicators* (January), 1965, iii-x; (September), 1965, 2-22; (November), 1965, 1-38; (December), 1965, 21-38.

3. Hearings on S 1606. National Health Program. US Senate Committee on Education and Labor, 79th Congr, Second Sess, 1946.

4. A Policy Statement on the Role of Government Tax Funds in Problems of Health Care. *Bulletin of the New York Academy of Medicine* XLI (July), 1965, 795-796. A more specific spelling out of objectives is contained in the American Public Health Association's two policy statements, Medical care in a national health program, *American Journal of Public Health* 34:1252-1256 (December), 1944; and The quality of medical care in a national health program, *Medical Care in Transition.* PHS Publication 1128, 1:17-43, 1964.

5. For some of the other issues which could not be dealt with in this paper see chapter 5 above.

6. The impressive statement that in 1963 no less than 70.3% of the civilian population had some form of hospital expense coverage while 63% had surgical coverage conceals the fact that for some sections of the population these percentages were very much lower. Families with incomes of less than $2,000 were covered only to the extent of 34%, while the nonwhite percentage was only

46% against a white percentage of 74. Coverage in the South was much lower than in other parts of the country. These figures are derived from the national household interview surveys. The Health Insurance Association of America places the national averages slightly higher. (Reed LS: The extent of health insurance coverage in the United States. Research Rep No 10. Social Security Administration, 1965.) See also Lawrence PS, Fuchsberg RR: Medical Care and Family Income. *Health, Education, and Welfare Indicators* (May), 1964, XXI-XXIV.

7. Reed LS, and Hanft RS: National Health Expenditures. *Social Security Bulletin* (January), 1966, 11.

8. For an evaluation of health needs of children, see Health of Chidlren of School Age. Children's Bureau Publication No 427, 1964.

9. Ball RM: Health insurance for people aged 65 and over: First steps in administration. *Social Security Bulletin* (February), 1966, 6.

10. Reed LS, Hanft RS: op cit, 11. Since the above was written, the Social Security Administration has estimated that total health expenditures in 1965-1966 amounted to $42.96 billions, or 6% of GNP. Merriam IC: Social welfare expenditures, 1965-1966. *Social Security Bulletin* (December), 1966, 16.

11. Training Health Service Workers. Proceedings of the Department of Labor. Department of Health, Education and Welfare Conference on Job Development and Training for Workers in Health Services (February), 1966. Washington, DC: Government Printing Office, 1966.

12. A convenient compilation of the various reports is contained in Anderson, OW: Influence of social and economic research on public policy in the health field: A review, in health services research *I. Milbank Memorial Fund Quarterly,* Vol XLIV, No 3 (July), 1966, Part II. See also Closing the gaps in the availability and accessibility of health services, The 1965 conference. New York Academy of Medicine. *Bulletin of the New York Academy of Medicine,* Vol 41, No 12 (December), 1965; and Heselkorn, F (ed), *Mothers-at-Risk, Perspectives in Social Work.* Vol 1, No 1, Adelphi University, Graduate School of Social Work, 1966.

13. Cf Burney, LE: The University and Community Health Services. *American Journal of Public Health.* 56,3:394-399 (March), 1966. See also Association of American Medical Colleges. *Medical Education in a Changing Society,* 1965. Published also as Part 2, Journal of Medical Education 40:1 (January), 1965.

14. Harris, R: Annals of legislation: Medicare. *The New Yorker* (July 3, 9, 16, and 23), 1966.

15. Falk, IS: Medicare: Where do we go from here? *Modern Hospitals* (June), 1966.

16. Terry, L: The complex world of modern public health. *American Journal of Public Health.* 54,2:189-195 (February), 1964.

17. Trussell, RE: The quality of medical care as a challenge to public health. *Ibid* 55,2:173-182 (February), 1965.

# PART 4
# POLICIES FOR TOMORROW

# 7    Is Health Insurance the Answer?

One can assume that in a symposium honoring Dr. Isidore S. Falk the words "health insurance" must refer not to private but to compulsory governmental health insurance, of which he has for so long been a powerful advocate. But the term "health insurance" is, as so often pointed out, itself misleading. The systems which have been developed all over the world certainly do not insure health. Some have suggested "sickness insurance" as being more accurate, but even that is ambiguous. What most of them do is to insure against the costs of medical treatment, and one is tempted to think that a more accurate name for our own venture into health insurance would be "Medicost," rather than "Medicare."

Essentially, health insurance is a method of spreading the costs of medical care, broadly or narrowly interpreted, over as large a proportion of the group at risk as possible. It is one device for removing all, or part, of the financial barrier to the receipt of medical care and health services. One would have thought that the case for using this device would have been so obvious that the United States would have long ago followed the example of other countries and instituted a health insurance system.[1] I still remember my astonishment when I arrived in this country in 1926, a wide-eyed student eager to learn about the social institutions of the United States, to find that apart from workmen's compensation there was no form of social insurance in effect, and that any such institution was regarded as something possibly appropriate for effete and unprogressive Europeans but certainly not needed by self-reliant and wealthy Americans. Even with the onset of

Presented at a symposium at the Yale Medical School in honor of Dr. Isidore S. Falk, and reprinted by permission from the *American Journal of Public Health*, Vol LIX, No 1, Part II (January 1969), 9-18.

the Depression, which turned men's minds to consideration of ways of assuring income maintenance, it was unemployment insurance, and to a lesser degree old-age insurance—but not health insurance—that attracted professional discussion and attention.

## The Movement for Health Insurance

In fact, of course, there had been earlier interest in health insurance. In 1912, National Health Insurance had been one of the major planks in Theodore Roosevelt's Progressive Party; organized social workers had made studies and proposals; several states had introduced and debated compulsory health insurance bills, and even the AMA had appeared to approve the principles embodied in some of these bills. Anne and Herman Somers have reminded us that as late as 1917 the AMA, when adopting a resolution concerning the principles that a proper health insurance system should include, stated "the time is present when the profession should study earnestly to solve the questions of medical care that will arise under various forms of social insurance. Blind opposition, indignant repudiation, bitter denunciation of these laws is worse than useless: it leads nowhere and it leaves the profession in a position of helplessness as the rising tide of social development sweeps over it."[2] One can only say "Amen!"

And "amen" in another sense it was! The war came, and when it was over the AMA, responding to the adverse reactions of state medical societies, declared its formal opposition to any plan of compulsory contributory insurance operated or controlled by government. The social workers turned their attention to the acquisition of professional status, stressed clinical service and casework and spent their energies on the absorption of Freudian principles that seemed to offer a basis for a unique, identifiable professional service. Until the Depression, social policy in general was neglected by them. Nor were matters helped by the stance of organized labor, which might have been expected to lead a movement for social insurance. For it was not until 1932 that the AFL formally withdrew its opposition to social insurance, and then only on condition that the costs be carried by the employer. Interest in the subject was kept alive only through the work of a few scholars (such as Rubinow or Armstrong), and the individuals associated with both the American Association for Social Security and the American Association for Labor Legislation.

Even the farsighted Committee on the Costs of Medical Care, 1927-1932 (with which I. S. Falk was prominently associated), while it recommended, in its majority report, financing through comprehensive

144

group payment, placed its reliance on voluntary action and refrained from recommending compulsory public health insurance. In subsequent years the spectacular growth of private (profit and nonprofit) health insurance seemed to promise that voluntary action might indeed be the answer.

The next opportunity for action came in 1934-1935 but the Committee on Economic Security did not include any proposals for health insurance in the proposed social security legislation, reportedly because it was felt by the Administration that to include so controversial a plan would have endangered the other, extremely important, old-age and unemployment-insurance provisions.

We are all familiar with the subsequent story: the efforts to enact federal health insurance (especially in the immediate postwar years), the gradual whittling down of the objectives—until we find ourselves, in 1965, regarding the passage of a limited health insurance measure for the aged as a great victory. To the extent that it is the *premier pas qui coute,* the 1965 legislation is of course an important milestone, the more important because of the very violence of the opposition. And yet from a broader perspective there may be less cause for rejoicing, for some of the price that was paid involved compromises that may make future progress more difficult. [3]

## The Achievements of Social Insurance

I have always been a great proponent of social insurance, and regard it as one of the major social inventions. It effected the transition from reliance on charity or grudging, and often degrading, public aid to a system of rights to socially assured income in the event of specific occurrences. It did so by linking the bestowal of rights to the concept of insurance, a thoroughly respectable and respected institution. So successfully was this done that today it is difficult to get students to realize that before 1935 in this country, not only was it a problem of getting the voters, as a group, to accept the fact that giving old or unemployed people the right to cash payments without undergoing a means test would not undermine the very basis of our capitalist free enterprise system, but it was also necessary to persuade the potential beneficiaries that there was nothing wrong or shameful about accepting such payments. The word "insurance" performed a very useful social function.

But social insurance has done more than this. It has proved to be a very effective method of raising money to finance welfare programs. People seem much more willing to pay taxes if they feel that they are going to benefit personally and directly from the expenditures. There is another side to this coin, of course, for we must never forget that it was the social insurance tax systems with their provision for employer withholding and their acceptability to workers which opened the eyes of treasuries to the fact that it was indeed possible to tax low-income receivers. Politicians have not been blind to this fiscal advantage of social insurance. In 1925, contributory old-age pensions in England were enacted by a Conservative government that was under great pressure to liberalize the noncontributory income-tested old-age pension system. Similarly it is not, I think, by accident that recently the governor of New York, faced with mounting costs of Medicaid, has become a most active proponent of compulsory health insurance.

In somewhat broader terms, contributory insurance also appears to provide some check on irresponsible liberalizations. The linkage of benefits and taxes has undoubtedly served up to now as a useful control in a world where competition for the taxpayer's dollar is intense. Finally, as its scope has widened (and coverage in terms of people had to be fairly broad even initially, in the interests of spreading the risk), social insurance has served as a socially cohesive force. It is not a program solely for "the poor." From the first a cross section of wage earners has been covered, thereby including the upper working-class groups, and increasingly the middle classes have also been included. Involvement of the direct interest of the middle classes has prevented social insurance from deteriorating into a program for the poor, for whom, alas, it often seems to be felt that anything is good enough. In a world that is increasingly subject to divisive forces, social insurance has stressed solidarity and mutuality of interest.

## Problems in Using Social Insurance for Health Services

So long as it was confined to dealing with loss or interruption of income, and to the making of cash payments, this instrument performed remarkably well. It has been essentially a mechanism for collecting funds and paying them out in specified contingencies. There have of course been problems and troublesome policy issues but they have proved manageable. There have been administrative problems in determining the occurrence of the risk insured against; for example, what is involuntary unemployment? When has a man retired? How the degree of disability that is held to prevent a man from working can be assessed? And there have been policy issues: who should be covered? What level of benefits should be payable? How should the costs be allocated among the covered population, their employers, and the general taxpayer?

These problems have been difficult enough but they are simple in comparison to those faced when social insurance is used to deal with the financial barriers to the receipt of services. Services have to be rendered by professionals whose responsible cooperation with the program is essential. When cash payments are made, it has proved possible to hire mainly nonprofessional staffs and use machines to check eligibility and calculate payments, even when the benefit formulas and the rules governing eligibility are extremely complicated. The criteria and formulas are highly objective, call for the exercise of minimal discretion, and their application rests in the hands of the public administrator. Where payment for services is the objective, organized professionals must first be induced to render these services to the insured. This is a matter partly of determining rates of remuneration acceptable to both the profession and the wider community, and partly of determining other conditions of employment to which professionals attach importance. The extent to which services were in fact rendered is attested to by the professionals or purveyors of service rather than by the administrator who, in effect, is underwriting all or part of a bill whose size is out of his direct control, and who depends on the professionals' competence and integrity.

Again, when making cash payments in the event of interruption of income, a dollar is a dollar. At any given time every dollar received by a beneficiary buys as much as that received by any other. Even changes over time in the value of the dollar have not proved impossible to adjust to; with services, however, the problem of variable quality arises. One then has to face the question whether the government, as operator of the system, has any responsibility for ensuring that the services received by its insured, for which it is paying, are indeed of minimally acceptable quality. In some cases the services may not be available at all and the system may be charged with deception for collecting contributions to pay for services that do not exist.

There is yet a third complication. In social insurance systems dealing with income maintenance, the question of how much of the taxpayer's income is to be devoted to this end (income transfers) can be openly debated and controlled by legislative decisions on eligibility rules and benefit formulas. The global costs of any given combination of these can be estimated with a high degree of reliability so that rational choices are possible and, once made, the administrator can control them. When it is a matter of paying for services, cost (i.e., the

147

taxpayer's bill) is affected not only by the decisions of individual practitioners and purveyors of care as to how much service is to be rendered but also by the prices charged by professionals and institutional suppliers, and by the efficiency or inefficiency of the organizational arrangements for the delivery of services.

There is one final difference in the application of social insurance to the problem of income maintenance and its application to the problem of health services. All social insurance systems contain eligibility criteria. Only those persons who have been "covered" for some specified period, or have paid some specified amount of taxes, or are related in some defined way to the insured person are eligible for benefits. This limitation of access to the program may make sense in a cash payment system (although we often carry the exclusions too far). As an example, if the system exists to replace income from work, then one needs some proof that the claimant was indeed normally working and the eligibility rules aim to test this and to eliminate the voluntarily unemployed. But once it is realized that the function of eligibility rules is to keep people out (i.e., to exclude), one may ask whether this concept is appropriate to a health service system where surely one wishes to exclude nobody who is in need of health services.

## Limited Use of Compulsory Health Insurance in the United States

It is perhaps not surprising that most countries, notably including our own, have first conceived of the problem in the health services as being one of removing the financial barrier. Even so, it has proved impossible to escape the problem of ensuring professional cooperation; in most countries the history of health insurance is replete with disputes between the authorities and the medical professions as to rates and methods of pay, and conditions of employment.[4]

### Removing the Financial Barrier

So far, we have not been very effective in using health insurance to remove the financial barrier. In the first place the coverage, in terms of population, is very restricted. The history of the postwar movement for health insurance is one of gradual retreat from the goal of almost universal coverage, as embodied in the early Wagner-Murray-Dingell bills, to coverage of the narrower group of the aged. Given the strength of the opposition, the 1951 decision to concentrate on the aged was probably inevitable. Their plight, in terms of need for health services and limited income with which to pay for them, could be demonstrated. The inability of private insurance to deal with the problem was becoming daily more evident, even to the insurance companies themselves. An effectively operating instrument, namely OASDI, was available, and the aged were numerous and had votes.

From a longer range point of view, of course, this concentration on the aged makes no sense. If the nation is unwilling to open the doors to needed health services for everyone, a different priority would seem obvious. A powerful case could be made for beginning at the other end of the life span and removing the barriers to health services for children. The national interest in having a healthy and productive labor force would alone argue for this, quite apart from other considerations. Perhaps even now we may hope that some ingenious mind will invent some way to reverse the concept of paid-up insurance as now applied to the aged in Title 18A and to provide postpaid insurance so that children can have health insurance protection *before* they enter what is now an almost universal contributory insurance system. Assuming certain changes in our present health insurance system, which I shall later suggest, this would surely be a better way of ensuring at least minimal health care for children rather than, as now, leaving them to the uncertain outcome of Medicaid developments.

I also suggest that we should not be too surprised at the recent reaction against Medicaid on the part of both Congress and the states. In my judgment, Title 19 attempted to achieve too much, too fast. To my knowledge, no other grant-in-aid program has ever been so completely open-ended or left the federal taxpayer so strongly committed to pay a bill the size of which he could in no way control. No other federal grant-in-aid program has ever contained so many standards and requirements for state programs; all these standards and requirements *aimed at wider coverage and increased service,* and carried the penalty of loss of existing federal grants if the states did not conform by specified dates. In any case, the objective of providing needed health services for all children through Medicaid will always be thwarted by the fact that everything depends on state action and whatever service is provided will reflect differences in states' resources and interests. If we are serious about providing for children with at least minimal adequacy, we shall have to look to federal action.

The inclusion of children and aged in federal health insurance would leave the productive age groups unprovided for. It is difficult to forecast the extent to which they will be able to meet the problem of health costs through private insurance. My own guess is that we shall increasingly find, as medical care costs rise, that private insurance will have a harder and harder selling job, and will find it difficult to cover an acceptable percentage of the ever-increasing medical bill. If this is so, we must expect pressure to extend federal health insurance to other adult groups. It seems obvious that Medicare will soon be extended to additional social security beneficiaries. The same arguments that were compelling for the age 65-and-over group apply equally to the disabled and to early retirees. Nor will it be easy in the years ahead to resist the claims of survivor beneficiaries whose incomes are, for the most part, limited.

I said earlier that we have not been very effective in using social insurance to remove the financial barrier to health care, in part because we limit coverage. However, in the immediate future the task of making health insurance more adequate (in the sense of doing the job it was devised to do more effectively) will be more important than extending coverage to more people. As a method of removing the financial barrier to access to needed health services, Medicare has two gross defects.

First, it still leaves the insured person with a sizable medical bill over and above his annual premium, because of the provisions for deductibles and coinsurance, and because of the leeway in Title 18B which permits doctors to charge what they think the traffic will bear over and above the reimbursable "reasonable and customary" charges. So far as deductibles and coinsurance are concerned, justification is apparently based on the assumption that people have an inordinate appetite for medical care and hospitalization, and this appetite must be checked. It is evidently also assumed that one cannot trust the professionals whose decisions govern whether a patient shall go to hospital or undergo specific tests or procedures. These assumptions need to be tested by research.

Admittedly there is a real problem of ensuring responsible use of a service that, apart from the premium, would be free. But an intelligent society would surely seek controls that do not have the undesirable consequences of forcing the patient to bear a sizable share of the bill over and above what he pays by way of a premium. Increasing efforts must be made to enlist more professional cooperation and self-policing. The experiences of nongovernmental prepaid comprehensive health plans with such controls must be more carefully studied, especially because these lend themselves to experimentation more readily than does a national program.

The limited financial protection of the patient, due to the physician's freedom to collect from him more than he will be reimbursed for, will be especially difficult to change. It was presumably part of the price paid for physicians' participation in the program. Perhaps we have to await a new generation of doctors whose professional training, we may hope, will include a far broader and more socially oriented concept of professional ethics.

### Selective Reimbursements not Service

The second shortcoming of contemporary health insurance is its selectivity about the reimbursable types of treatment and the places where treatment is received. This unfortunate item-by-item approach to the payment of medical costs is further complicated by the existence of two separate and confusing reimbursement systems, parts A and B. From the financial point of view, this policy of reimbursing for some items only, again leaves some patients with sizable bills and limits the extent to which health insurance removes the financial barrier.

The major thrust of reform should be directed to removal of this selective reimbursement system for even more compelling reasons than the financial one. The present reimbursement system interposes an unnecessary barrier to the planning of appropriate courses of treatment, distorts professional advice by considerations of finance, and influences the extent to which patients can or will act on the advice given. Above all, this item-by-item method of meeting the costs of medical care, coupled with the exclusion of some items, fosters fragmentation of service, which is the outstanding weakness of our present system for the delivery of health services.

Thus I would urge that the first priority for effective utilization of health insurance is insistence on comprehensiveness of service coverage. This is even more crucial than removal of deductibles and coinsurance, and it is more important than extending coverage to additional population groups, even though the latter is desirable and politically feasible.

I said earlier that the dimensions of the problem of assuring health services for all are broader than the mere removal of the financial barrier. Availability of facilities, supporting services and personnel, assurance of high quality of service, and economy in the use of funds and resources—all call for urgent attention. To what extent may we expect the health insurance system as such to grapple with them? Certainly not all health insurance systems have accepted responsibility in these areas. Between 1911 and 1948 the British health insurance system limited itself essentially to paying bills. Availability, quality, and use of resources were none of its concern. Health insurance systems in other countries either have been slow to act in these difficult areas or have done so only with reluctance. Nor is it surprising that initially the question of availability and quality of care should have been relatively neglected by the health insurance authorities. For in the 1880's when

Germany began to develop its system, and the early 1900's when Britain and other countries were developing their systems, the scientific revolution in medicine had scarcely begun. What passed for acceptable professional service then available. Probably people in general were less aware of the potentials of good health services and of the difference between good and poor quality service. We live today in a scientific and technological era, and people's sights have been raised. Today, people will not be satisfied with the mere removal of the financial barrier, and we can no longer neglect the organizational and related problems that have been brought about by the scientific and technological revolutions.

*Supply and availability of personnel and facilities.* Some health insurance authorities have, however, made efforts to deal with problems of supply and availability by building and operating their own hospitals, clinics, convalescent homes, and other facilities in which their own staffs provide group care. I do not see us following this pattern, at least not until the population coverage of health insurance is much wider than it now is. Parallel delivery systems, one for the limited group of the aged that is insured and another for the noninsured, would perpetuate and strengthen our already undesirable two-class health-service system. Such a policy would be met by insistence by the medical profession on free choice of doctor, a demand which appears to have considerable support from the population at large. We here may recognize that realistically—even when the financial barrier is removed —free choice of doctor is largely an illusion because choice is restricted to the selection of the primary physician, and free choice of institution is limited by the availability of beds and the admission policies of individual hospitals. However, the idea of free choice has broad popular appeal. Our hope is that the health insurance system will prove flexible enough to give full support to groups providing comprehensive high quality care and that in time the superiority of this method will become evident and win out in competition. But here again there will be need for both careful evaluative studies and wide dissemination of the results.

Other countries such as Sweden have responded to the problem of supply and availability by direct provision by government, rather than by the health insurance system, of certain types of institutions such as hospitals. These are open to all on either a free or a nominal charge basis and when charges are made, the health insurance authorities purchase service on behalf of their members. I suspect that this will be the more probable trend in the United States. The health insurance system will remain largely a financing mechanism but government will be heavily involved in the construction of facilities that are either publicly operated (directly or through public corporations) or privately operated under increasingly close public supervision. Government will also play a large role in assuring an adequate supply of needed personnel through subsidizing education and training.

*Quality of care.* It already seems evident that the health insurance administrators in the United States cannot escape some degree of involvement in another area of concern, quality of care. A major step in this direction has been taken in the formal conditions of participation laid down for certain types of institutions and providers of technical services. Quality control will, however, be easier to achieve for institutional care than for practitioner services. In both cases, two needs are apparent. To the extent that the instrument used is accreditation (or licensing) and consultation, we must develop stronger and better staffed state (and even local) health departments. There is also a need for much more research into measures of, and methods of control over, quality.

*Economical use of resources.* In regard to the problem of the economical use of health resources, we may indeed expect major leadership to come from the health insurance authorities. Inefficient or uneconomic resource use by a health insurance system shows up immediately in increased costs that at once become visible and onerous through increased contributions or taxes. We may therefore expect that the administrators of Medicare will increasingly chafe under the restrictions imposed by the preamble to Title 18, whereby there is a disclaimer of any effort by government to interfere in the methods by which health services are delivered and administered. I am also sure that the Congress will look with increasing favor on investigations into the extent to which the methods of rendering services, and the organization and administration of medical institutions, involve unnecessary costs. There is already an awareness of the extent to which reimbursement formulas can affect costs. The amendments of 1967 authorize the Secretary of HEW to experiment with various methods of reimbursement to physicians and organizations "that would provide incentives for limiting the costs of the programs while maintaining quality care." Once again a vast new field for demonstration and research has opened up. The Medicare administrators will also possess a rich store of data which will facilitate sophisticated statistical comparisons of the performance of both institutions and practitioners. As the arrangements for determining reasonable costs and charges are renegotiated, the purveyors of health services will have to be prepared to answer some awkward questions.

At the same time there is a danger in sole reliance on the health insurance authorities to press for more efficient methods of delivery, for their main concern will be financial. It is not always the case that the method which saves money is the one that renders service in the most desirable way. Many of the changes that one might envisage, such as a central data bank or a centralized community-operated ambulance or laboratory service, would meet the demands of both economy and better service. But from such reading as I have done, it does not seem indisputably clear that group practice, although it renders better service, is necessarily cheaper than solo practice. The need therefore is for vigilance, a vigilance that must come from two sources. On the one hand we need more knowledge from nonofficial sources about what is happening; here the responsibility is clearly on the universities, medical schools, and research centers. On the other hand, we need to make more provision for representation of the consumers in the administrative structure of our health insurance system. Up to now we have been extraordinarily fortunate in the caliber and sense of public interest of the federal administrators, but they are in a difficult position and are subject to heavy pressure from the organized purveyors of health services. The administrators need an organized constituency on the other side, if only as a countervailing force. It is neither fair nor reasonable to expect them to carry the entire responsibility for protecting the interests of the consumers of health services. High on my agenda for making health insurance a more effective instrument in this country is provision for more effective user representation and influence.

## Future Directions and the Role of Research

Like Dr. Falk,[5] I do not see us moving rapidly toward a national health service. I still believe a free national health service to be the most effective instrument yet devised for assuring universal access to the full range of comprehensive health services; even while saying this, I recognize that national services also have some unsolved problems. However, the very size and diversity of this country suggest that such a system would be difficult for us to organize and administer. At the same time we must not forget that we do in fact have a national health

154

service—for veterans. Perhaps we could start by developing a national health service for children.

It took Great Britain over 30 years of experience with a much more extensive health insurance system than ours to get to the point of switching to a free health service; even then the change might not have come had not the war and the blitz thrown the inefficiencies and inadequacies of the existing system into relief.[6] The rising costs of health care may propel us faster than I now anticipate into a radical reorganization of our health delivery systems. However, unlike the British, we are affluent and can tolerate a lot of waste. Organized medicine in this country is more resistant to change, but even here there are some faint signs of recognition of the changed world.

Much depends too, on what happens under Medicaid. The current adverse reactions should not blind us to the potential of this program. Because it is a state (and even a locally) influenced program it will lend itself to experimentation. It will be of the utmost importance that these experiments be recorded and evaluated. We may indeed find that here and there Medicaid programs are developing which offer comprehensive care under nonoffensive conditions that may compare very favorably with what the health insurance system has been able to deliver. The important thing will be to make effective use of the much vaunted experimentation potential offered by our numerous states and political subdivisions—"effective use" means capturing and recording the results and disseminating widely the knowledge thus gained.

As he looks back on his long and richly productive professional career, Isidore Falk must have many reasons for satisfaction. Health insurance, for which he fought so long and so valiantly, is no longer a dirty word but an established institution. I have no doubt that in a few years young students will be describing it as "the American way" of handling a problem, as they now do with OASI! Both the changing public attitude about what is expected from a health system and the vast scientific and technological changes that have affected the health services have created new problems that are more complicated than can be dealt with by a health insurance system alone. Today we have to ask what the role of health insurance is in a complex of institutions and arrangements for the provision of health services to all. Even now we can foresee a considerably larger role for health insurance than it now plays.

Perhaps even more than in the enactment of a health insurance system, Falk must feel a deep satisfaction in the increasing attention paid by scholars (medical and nonmedical experts alike) to research in the health services field. Once almost a lone wolf, at any rate a member

155

of a tiny pack, he is today one of the outstanding leaders of a sizable and ever-growing group of men and women whose work—and this is the important point—is directed toward the solution of the health service problems of the real world. When one asks in which direction we should move, one finds the first essential is to know more about what is happening and about what works and what does not.

Despite disturbing signs of growing irrationality in the world I still believe, as does Myrdal,[7] that knowledge is a powerful force for bringing about change and reform. I believe this is Dr. Falk's credo, too. It is because he has asked questions of relevance to the functioning of our health services and because he has helped to find some of the answers, either directly or through those he has influenced, that we honor him today—a scholar whose work has affected public policy.

## Notes

1. For a list of contemporary Health Insurance Systems see Social Security Programs Throughout the World, 1967. US Department of Health, Education and Welfare, Social Security Administration, Office of Research and Statistics, Washington DC: Government Printing Office, 1967.

2. Somers HM, Somers AR: *Medicare and the Hospitals, Issues and Prospects.* Washington, DC, The Brookings Institution, 1967, 2.

3. Burns EM: *Policy Decisions Facing the United States in Financing and Organizing Health Care.* Public Health Report 81,8:675-683 (August 1966).

4. See, for instance, International Social Security Association: *Relations Between Social Security Institutions and the Medical Profession.* Eleventh General Meeting, Report IV, Geneva, Switzerland, The Association, 1953; Hogarth J: *The Payment of the General Practitioner; Some European Comparisons.* Oxford, England, Pergamon, and New York, Macmillan, 1963.

5. Falk IS: Medical Care and Social Policy. *American Journal of Public Health* 55,4:526 (April 1965).

6. Titmuss RM: *Problems of Social Policy.* London, HM Stationery Office, and Ontario, Canada, Longmans, Green, 1950.

7. Myrdal G: The social sciencies and their impact on society. Stein HD (ed): *Social Theory and Social Invention.* Cleveland, Ohio: The Press of Case-Western Reserve University, 1968.

# 8 A Critical Review of National Health Insurance Proposals

It is evident that within the next few years we shall see some major extensions of governmentally supported insurance against the costs of health services. Even the American Medical Association (AMA) and the insurance companies see the handwriting on the wall and are coming up with their own proposals. The mounting insistence that there should be further governmental involvement in this area stems from two major influences. First, the very existence of Medicare has demonstrated that public compulsory health insurance is feasible. Despite its many well-known weaknesses, Medicare obviously has brought considerable financial relief to, and broadened access to health services for, many millions of the aged, and it is popular. Inevitably, there is growing pressure to extend a similar service to those whose economic circumstances differ little, if at all, from those of the mass of the aged. If aged social security beneficiaries, why not disabled beneficiaries? If the disabled, why not survivor families?

We are already seeing, too, criticism of the limited scope of the types of health services covered by the insurance program. Why exclude preventive check-ups, or drugs, or certain other components of comprehensive care? If paid-up insurance is feasible for hospital and institutional care, why it is not equally applicable to physicians' services?

Even more influential in stimulating a demand for an extension of compulsory health insurance is the impact on all sections of the population, and not merely the aged, of the sharply rising costs of health services, so especially pronounced since 1965. These increased

Based on a paper presented as the Keynote Address at the Group Health Institute, Honolulu, Hawaii, May 25, 1970 and published by permission of the Group Health Association of America in *HSMHA Health Reports,* LXXXVI, No 2 (February 1971), 111-120.

costs are reflected in a continuing upward trend in the premiums charged by private health insurers, both profit and nonprofit, or in some curtailment of benefits so that the contribution these institutions can make to moderating the financial burden on even middle-class families will inevitably decline. They may indeed be in danger of pricing themselves out of the market.

The result has been a flood of bills and proposals and plans. The AMA has made proposals[1]; so have the Equitable and the Aetna insurance companies.[2] Governor Nelson A. Rockefeller has again introduced a health insurance bill in New York[3], and the Committee on Human Resources of the National Governors' Conference has endorsed a system of universal health insurance[4] following the general lines of the earlier Rockefeller bill. The AFL-CIO has made some proposals, now embodied in the Griffiths bill.[5] The Committee for National Health Insurance (CNHI), formed by the late Walter Reuther, has been intensively working on a proposal for national health insurance, which, under the title of the Health Security Act, has now been introduced by Senator Kennedy.[6] Among other bills are those sponsored by Representative Dingell,[7] jointly by Representative Fulton and Senator Fannin,[8] and by Senator Javits.[9] Organizations such as the American Public Health Association also have committees working on a program for national health services.

It is obvious that space alone will preclude a detailed consideration of each and all of these numerous schemes. In any event, a detailed comparison of their features would be extremely repetitious and boring. I propose instead to discuss some of the more crucial features and problems of any health insurance system and to examine how these are dealt with by some of these plans.

As we consider them, it is well to bear in mind the objectives to which almost everyone gives lip service. What we are seeking, I assume, is a program that assures universal access to comprehensive and continuous health services of high quality, delivered under circumstances that are convenient, comfortable, and dignified and in a manner that is efficient and economical. Several features of current proposals bear directly on the attainment of these objectives.

## A Voluntary or Compulsory Plan?

A number of proposals, notably those of the AMA as embodied in the Fulton bill, the earlier Fannin-Fulton bills, and those of the insurance companies, envisage a vast expansion of voluntary insurance through the use of tax incentives. These incentives would take the form of a tax credit—the amount would vary either with the level of adjusted gross income or, as with the Fulton (AMA) bill, the level of tax liability—equal to some percentage of the costs of purchasing a qualified insurance policy. Receivers of very low income would get government certificates enabling them to purchase such a policy.

In contrast, the proposals of Governor Rockefeller and the National Governors' Conference, Senator Javits, the AFL-CIO (Griffiths bill), the Dingell bill, and the Kennedy (CNHI) bill provide for a compulsory system whereby both employers and workers would be required to pay social insurance taxes to support the system. There is also an element of compulsion in the proposals of the Aetna insurance company, which rely on an extension of fringe benefits to cover a large proportion of workers. They would penalize an employer for not broadening existing health benefits plans to the required extent by cutting in half the tax deduction he could claim for his contributions to his existing plan. The Griffiths, Kennedy, and Javits bills envisage a contribution from the general revenues toward program costs, while the governors admit the possible necessity for such a contribution if employee and employer taxes are not to exceed some reasonable ceiling.

It seems highly doubtful whether, even as thus subsidized, the voluntary approach would ensure universal coverage or effectively remove the financial barrier. Quite apart from the problem of reaching and enrolling those who normally pay no tax or are not employed, which is admitted by the sponsors, it seems unlikely that many millions of families who are not now insured or adequately insured could be induced to lay out the sizable sums necessary to purchase adequate coverage. Dr. Russell B. Roth, speaking for the AMA, has estimated that "a package providing minimal benefits which can justify a description of comprehensive protection will cost something like $700 a year for an average family." Yet to increase the share of the premium provided by the tax credit would vastly increase the cost of the program.

The Pettengill or Aetna proposal places heavy reliance on an extension and liberalization of fringe benefits as the method of enrolling the vast majority of workers, and provides a second subsidized program for the long-period unemployed, the near-poor whose employers do not provide group medical coverage, and those who are uninsurable because of poor health. Incidentally, the groups not covered by employer fringe-benefit plans will be larger than this. For these groups it is proposed that federal action should encourage the states to develop a system of uniform health insurance benefits to be operated by a reinsurance plan underwritten by all carriers and for which the poor would be covered free, the near-poor would make a

159

contribution varying inversely with adjusted income, while the uninsurable would pay a fraction of a premium that would reflect their high claims costs. The difference between the needed premiums and those charged against these three groups would be carried by the state, which would receive between 65 and 90% reimbursement from the federal government. Yet when we recall the many claims on state resources and the unwillingness of many states to undertake further expenditures under Medicaid and existing health programs, it seems highly unlikely that any plan which relies on state action for the coverage of those not benefiting from fringe-benefit health programs can hope to succeed.

A further objection to proposals that aim to make it possible, through subsidies from the government, for low-income receivers to buy insurance is that it perpetuates and indeed extends income testing. For the proponents of this approach recognize that a uniform subsidy for each insured person such as that offered under title XVIIIB of the Social Security Act will not meet the problem. Many people need a subsidy of much more than 50%. Yet the alternative (namely, to vary the subsidy with the size of a person's income or, as in the Pettengill or Aetna proposals, to have separate and variable subsidies for the poor, the near-poor, and the uninsurable) is to perpetuate the kind of social divisiveness that is currently causing so much concern. It will also be far from administratively simple as people move from one classification to another (poor to near-poor to not poor, and vice versa) or as their incomes change or as efforts are made to avoid "notch" problems.

With the current euphoria about family assistance plans and negative income taxes, we are in danger of becoming a needs- or income-tested nation. We already have means tests for subsidized housing, school meals, surplus foods and food stamps, educational grants, day care, and other services. The Heineman commission[10] has estimated that a guarantee of a poverty-line income today would involve income supplements to some 24 million households. Do we want to add to the millions who must individually contact government and undergo a means test to secure some financial assistance? One of the most important questions of principle to be decided is whether any health services plan should involve income tests.

It should be noted, however, that the compulsory plans which take the form of a requirement to pay social insurance taxes also have to face the problem of coverage of those who either do not or cannot pay the specified taxes. The Griffiths, Javits, and Kennedy bills aim to minimize the deterrent to enrollment presented by a heavy wage tax by providing for a contribution to the scheme from the general revenues.

The public assistance population can indeed be covered by requiring states with or without a federal subsidy to take out insurance premiums on behalf of their caseloads, though with fluctuating loads due to turnover this will be no simple administrative task. But there still remains the problem of the millions of irregularly employed workers and of migrants and the like who are hard to catch for tax purposes.

The Griffiths and Kennedy bills, and apparently the Javits bill, provide what would seem to be the correct answer. They make all citizens and permanent residents of the United States eligible for the promised benefits, thus in effect separating the determination of eligibility from the financing of the program and leaving it to the tax collector to gather in as much revenue from the wage and payroll taxes as he can. This is a sharp break with the original insurance theory that the right to benefits should be dependent on having paid the necessary number of contributions or taxes, but it is questionable how far today we need to limit the right to access to health services by resorting to this ideology. Wage and payroll taxes can be defended independently as a rich source of revenue helping to support the program; they do not also have to be the determinant of benefit rights.

## The Role of Private Insurance Companies

The plans of the AMA, the insurance companies, Senator Javits, and Governor Rockefeller would utilize private insurance as the central agencies for developing and operating the programs. Even Governor Rockefeller's recent proposals for encouraging nonprofit medical corporations seem to assume that these corporations in turn will contract with insurance carriers.

In contrast, the Griffiths and Kennedy bills would bypass the private insurance system except apparently for the possibility, in the Kennedy bill, of their limited use as representatives of the providers of services.

It seems likely that in the immediate future no issue will be more central or more hotly debated than the role of private insurance in either a government-subsidized voluntary or a compulsory social insurance system. The advocates of the private insurers claim that their involvement is in keeping with American ideology. It maximizes the freedom of choice of the consumer and offers the advantages of private initiative and competition. But the involvement of private insurance also commits the program to the ideology of private insurance with its understandable preoccupation with fiscal considerations and its concern about strictly defined and specified benefits and the use of deductibles and coinsurance. (Incidentally, the Griffiths bill provides for copayment, as does the Javits bill for drugs.)

The necessity to conform to private insurance principles has two major disadvantages. First, cost considerations prevent any private plan from underwriting the entire range of health services. The Aetna plan recognizes this weakness and proposes an additional governmentally supported program of catastrophic insurance. But this, apart from the unlikelihood that it would be everywhere effective since it depends on state initiative and financial support, carries with it such heavy deductibles that it is unlikely to be of much assistance to the middle-class patient faced with heavy medical costs. And the addition of yet a third program creates an administrative monstrosity.

Second, and perhaps even more important, the resulting inclusion of only some health services perpetuates the fragmentation of care, which is everywhere deplored, while the existence of deductibles, copayment, and coinsurance discourages early utilization of health services, especially those of a preventive character.

Against the possible advantages of competition must be set the added costs of securing business, much of which will have to be written on an individual basis, and presumably an allowance for profit. These costs would be negligible or nonexistent in a compulsory publicly operated plan. Allowance must be made, too, for the lowered level of efficiency attributable to a multiplicity of plans and for the governmental costs of approving and policing the systems. Problems of accountability would be intensified, especially if the insurance carriers were permitted to offer a package of benefits different from those prescribed if "actuarially equivalent and equal in health value" (temporarily in the Rockefeller plan) or "equivalent and at no greater cost," as in the Javits bill, which also envisages contracting out by employers who provide fringe benefits of a type and level superior to the national plan in terms of actuarial and health care considerations.

It is indeed somewhat surprising that the insurance companies have not had some second thoughts about involvement in a program that would inevitably bring about a considerable measure of public control of their activities. For, given the magnitude of the expenditures and the public interest in medical care, government would be compelled to exercise some control over the way in which the private insurance companies were administering the vast amount of subsidized business that was being thrown to them. Minimum requirements for an acceptable or approved policy, prohibitions of discrimination against certain types of would-be insurers, the permissibility of merit rating, control of the reasonableness of premiums both for legally prescribed benefits and, as in the Javits bill, any supplementary benefits and the like would seem unavoidable.

Experience with private insurance agencies as intermediaries involved in the reimbursement of providers under Medicare gives little reason other than political considerations for continuing their use even in this more limited capacity. As many of us pointed out in 1965, it was not very reasonable to expect an agency competing for business from providers to develop a reputation for strict application of rules and regulations and keen scrutiny of charges and volume of service in the interests of keeping down costs, no part of which they had to pay. I submit that the mounting costs of Medicare have justified these gloomy prophecies.

Nevertheless, if the private insurance companies are not to be intimately involved in the organization and administration of the program, other more appropriate administrative bodies at the subfederal level must be utilized. Here, differences seem to turn on the role to be assigned to the states as against new regional bodies. Failing the assumption of organizing and administrative responsibilities by private health insurance companies, the Javits bill provides for the creation of national health insurance corporations operating as agencies for the federal government and also permits the states to conclude agreements with the federal government to administer, as agents, all or part of the program. The Griffiths bill provides for administration of the federal program through a group of regional administrations, which will be empowered to enter into contracts with providers of medical, dental, and hospital services and to carry out other extensive responsibilities. The Kennedy bill also contemplates a regional basis of administration under a federal health security board, although the states are given responsibilities for planning and coordinating health services but, it would seem, without any effective powers to enforce their policies.

Some critics who fear that regions are artificial constructs with no solid base of political or financial support would prefer to see the program administered by the states on the basis of contracts with the federal government, which *inter alia* would provide for the setting up of regions. It is argued in further support of this position that the states are already involved in a variety of important health services and are the only entities in a position to develop services additional to those financed by the basic plan.

Even a compulsory publicly administered program faces the necessity of defining the services it will finance or provide. Given the present shortage and maldistribution of manpower and facilities and the high costs of some of the more exotic procedures, no system can guarantee the complete range of possible services to everyone. Even the Griffiths and Kennedy bills, which offer perhaps the widest range of services, limit dental care to young persons and, in the Griffiths bill, to some categories of the poor. The literature and the proposals are full of references to "the basic health services" that a national program would guarantee. But of what do the basic services consist? Is it possible to define them without running up against the problem of the item-by-item approach ... the effect on comprehensiveness and continuity of having some services for which costs will be covered and some for which they won't? Is it possible to approach comprehensive coverage in stages, as the Javits, Governors' Conference, and Kennedy proposals (for dental services) suggest; if so, what should be included at each stage? Or should the policy rather be to make the distinction not on the basis of type of treatment or illness or timing but on giving priority for full service to certain population categories? Might it make more sense to aim first of all to cover all the health needs of children?

## The Effect on Service Delivery

Government, despite its growing financial commitment, hitherto has been reluctant to become involved in the structure, organization, and administration of health services. In the preamble to title XVIII of the Social Security Act, any such intention was expressly disclaimed: "Nothing in this title shall be construed to authorize any Federal officer or employee to exercise any supervision or control over the ... manner in which medical services are provided ... or to exercise any supervision or control over the administration ... of any institution, agency, or person." Thus government has deferred to the practices of private insurance not only by admitting them as intermediaries but also by adopting a reimbursement system on an item-by-item basis and such cost-controlling provisions as deductibles, copayment, and coinsurance. It has deferred to the medical profession by making no effort to encourage departure from solo practice or a fee-for-service method of remuneration. It has, with the notable exception of New York and a handful of other states, made no effort to control the proliferation of unnecessary facilities and underutilized specialized equipment or their inappropriate location, though encouragement has been given to voluntary planning ... but without teeth, presumably in deference to the hospital establishment.

This timidity is unlikely to last much longer. First, the rising costs of health services are now, thanks to Medicare and Medicaid, highly visible, and we have a growing body of data on a nationwide scale that permits sophisticated statistical analysis and comparison. The political undesirability of having to increase both social security taxes and appropriations from the general revenues, or to curtail promised benefits by increased deductibles or reduced services, or to narrow the groups of eligible people is propelling government into a concern for the causes of rising costs and a search for controls. On all sides today, it is admitted that a major cause of the costliness of health services is the nature of the delivery system itself. It is significant that the Administration's proposed addition of payments to health maintenance organizations under Medicare, which would presumably encourage a different type of delivery system, was put forward not as one might have hoped because it would improve the service received by the insured, but mainly because it was believed to save money.

In the second place, government no longer needs to be afraid of and subservient to the providers of health services. The prestige of the medical profession is not as high as it was, and its influence on public policy is correspondingly weaker. A more literate and sophisticated public is less impressed by the mystique of the physician and more likely to question his views. The organized medical profession has contributed to this decline in prestige. Its prolonged opposition to any social health insurance program, even for the aged, where the gap between need for care and ability to pay for it is so obviously large, has left a nasty taste in the national mouth. Even more destructive of the old image is the unfortuante impression that the medical profession is greedy and has taken advantage of the reimbursement provisions of Medicare and Medicaid to enrich itself. The profession can rightly claim that such antisocial behavior is characteristic of only a small minority of physicians. Yet the profession should take a lesson from the welfare field: abuse of that system by a few recipients has been sufficient to damn the entire welfare population as lazy, improvident, greedy, and unscrupulous. The famous case of the "relief recipient with a mink coat" still influences the public image of the welfare clientele.

Nor need government continue to be so squeamish about interfering in the way hospitals are organized and run. For with the growing dependence of the voluntary hospitals on public funds, the government is in a powerful position to exercise strong-arm financial pressures and to claim that receipt of public money implies conformity with public policy.

Thus both the need and the opportunity for government to become involved in the health services delivery system are much greater than they were even 10 years ago. What advantage do the various proposals now before us take of this situation?

All proponents of health insurance plans now proclaim their recognition of the fact that the problems besetting the health care industry cannot be resolved merely by making more money available for the purchase of care. They differ, however, in their identification of major problems, in the methods they propose for dealing with them, and in the extent to which they would use the health insurance system as a vehicle for bringing about change.

All proposals include provisions aiming to keep down costs. Some would limit charges by, for example, providing that fees cannot exceed the prevailing level of fees in the community (Aetna), or should not increase faster than the general price level (Secretary of Health, Education and Welfare), or that hospital costs should not increase out of proportion to general payroll increases in given areas (Governors' Conference), or provide for setting a limit to total annual program expenditures (Kennedy), or require conformity with professional fee schedules set by official regional councils (Rockefeller), or prescribe that total costs may not increase more rapidly than average wage levels (Javits). Several suggest that institutional reimbursement should be on the basis of a predetermined annual budget instead of the present cost-reimbursement system.

Most plans envisage the development of incentive reimbursement formulas offering rewards for efficiency and economy and better utilization. Indeed one gets the impression that incentive plans are the "in" thing now.

Recognizing that costs are affected not only by unit charges but also by the number of units of service rendered, most plans also contain provisions aiming to ensure economical utilization. The Griffiths bill would make the receipt of all professional services dependent on the order of a primary physician or dentist who alone would be directly remunerated. Aetna would require a review committee of qualified physicians passing on the necessity and appropriateness of services if a hospital were to be approved, and most of the other plans make provision for some form of peer review or utilization committee. In addition to the requirement of utilization committees in hospitals and skilled nursing homes, the Kennedy bill would provide for similar controls over the use of drugs and make only approved drugs reimbursable.

Space does not permit a listing, let alone an evaluation of the effectiveness, of the various cost-control measures. But a few doubts may be voiced. How feasible will it be to set limits to reimbursable costs by reference to general price or wage levels or prevailing fees? Haven't we tried prevailing fees already? How justified are the high hopes now being placed on incentive schemes? How much reliance can be placed on peer review of the professional performance of colleagues?

In any event, certain observations can be made about all these cost-controlling proposals. First, more attention is paid to controlling charges and volume of service of institutional providers than of practitioners. Second, in most plans—the Kennedy bill is perhaps an exception—the control of quality is given much less attention than the control of costs. For the control of quality, reliance usually is placed on the setting of standards for participating institutions and professionals— the Kennedy and Griffiths bills devote much attention to these—though it would seem that only the Javits and Kennedy bills provide for stricter relicensing provisions to offset obsolescence of professional knowledge and, in the Javits bill, for the possibility of national licensing standards. In some instances peer review is cited as a device for controlling quality. Third, all these cost-control measures are directed toward the performance of the individual provider. They could operate with no change in the existing costly and inefficient delivery system.

At this point we come to a major difference between the proposals; namely, in the extent to which measures to improve the delivery of services are envisaged as an integral part of the health insurance system itself. On the one hand the AMA and the insurance companies see any such measures as calling for quite independent programs. The AMA expressly states that it "would surely make no sense" to burden the insurance program with these responsibilities. Their disregard of the delivery problem is evident in the fact that they propose to perpetuate the present unsatisfactory dual program now found in parts A and B of Medicare. The Aetna proposals recognize the need for more and better arrangements for ambulatory care and for teamwork and group practice, but suggest only a separate program of federal grants to train physicians in primary care and in managing teams of professional and allied personnel together with a federal program of loan guarantees for construction of ambulatory care centers and loans (grants in poverty areas) for "set-up" costs.

In sharp contrast, the Javits, Kennedy, and Griffiths bills would use the financial leverage of the insurance system to bring about change. The Kennedy bill devotes much attention to the promotion of health service organizations stressing health maintenance and ambulatory care, which will undertake to provide, or arrange for, complete health care, or at least the complete range of health security services to an enrolled or local population. This care is to be provided through prepaid group practice or an approximation thereto. To this end, a health resources development account, financed ultimately by 5% of the sums in the trust fund, would be set up to administer a program of grants and loans for expansion or establishment, which would be available for both existing (up to 80% of costs) and new such organizations (up to 90%). In addition, there would be loans at 3%, in the same proportions, for capital construction.

Starting-up costs would be subsidized for the first five years. Additionally, special improvement grants would be made to public or other nonprofit agencies to assist them in establishing improved coordination and linkages with other providers of services, while organizations providing comprehensive ambulatory care would be given grants for improving records, establishing information retrieval systems, and purchasing equipment for various purposes. Reimbursement of the costs of certain services, such as those of nutrition personnel or social workers, would be made only if rendered by comprehensive health service organizations. The bill also provides that federal law will supersede state laws which restrict the development of prepaid group practice.

Concern about the delivery system is also seen in the duties and powers given to the health security board to strengthen health planning throughout the country, with emphasis first on the special needs for personnel, facilities, and organization that will be necessitated by the new service, and second on the continuing improvement of the capabilities for the effective delivery of health services.

The Javits bill also makes specific proposals for changing the delivery system. Title IV of this bill, subsequently introduced as a separate bill, includes a series of measures to encourage the development of local comprehensive health service systems based on primary service areas. Grants equal to 80% of the cost of planning and developing such systems would be offered, together with technical assistance, assumption of the difference between income and operating costs during the first five years, capital grants up to 80% of the nonfederal contributions under Title VI of the Public Health Service Act, a 50% grant plus a loan at 3% if no other assistance is given for modernization, rehabilitation, or construction of ambulatory centers, and a subsidy to keep interest down to 1% for the development of facilities operated as part of a group practice system. In addition, such systems would be permitted to retain up to two thirds of the difference between their actual costs per member and those of comparable groups in the community.

Finally, under the Javits bill, all providers entering into agreements or contracts to provide services must undertake to make continuing studies of the organization and delivery methods in their geographic areas and of possible improvements, and to take action, or to recommend action to the Secretary of Health, Education and Welfare, calculated to provide greater continuity and comprehensiveness and to control unnecessary utilization.

The Griffiths bill, to promote continuity of care and presumably economy, provides that all agreements between the administrators and professional providers shall be limited to primary physicians or dentists. Their remuneration, on a per capita basis, would be sufficient to permit them to provide or arrange and pay for the needed services of specialists and other licensed health professionals, who in turn could be remunerated on a salary, capitation, or fee-for-service basis. Similarly, agreements between short-term hospitals or groups of hospitals would provide sufficient reimbursement on a capitation basis to permit them to pay for skilled nursing home care, home health services, and rehabilitation services.

Part B of the Griffiths bill also provides for grants from the health insurance funds to hospitals, medical groups, nonprofit organizations, and consumer cooperatives—up to 75% of the cost of planning and developing comprehensive health service delivery systems. To assist in staffing the new comprehensive health service delivery systems, a small revolving loan fund is provided, while title VI of the Public Health Service Act is to be amended to give priority in authorized loans and grants for construction to such comprehensive plans.

The Griffiths bill assigns to the regional administrators the duty of making studies of the ways and means by which the quality of health care and the efficiency of its delivery may be improved in their regions. They are also required to allocate funds so as to "reasonably assure" the availability of needed services in all areas. Provision also is made for the appointment of regional consumer advisory committees, to be concerned with the delivery system in their areas, which are to be staffed by professionals who are competent in medical care administration and organization, planning, public health and epidemiology, statistics, and health education.

Two other health insurance proposals aim to deal with the delivery system. The Administration has recently proposed the addition of a new provision in title XVIII of the Social Security Act under which the aged can elect to join a "health maintenance organization," which will provide in the form of a guaranteed package all the promised Medicare benefits plus preventive services. These health maintenance organizations will be reimbursed on a capitation basis, and any savings through efficiency consistent with quality will go to the organization and the consumer. The Rockefeller bill aims to encourage group practice by permitting the formation of profitmaking professional health service corporations to render specified professional services, and to stimulate the growth of prepaid comprehensive care programs by providing for the formation of nonprofit medical corporations. The corporations would be empowered to provide medical services and to provide or arrange for any health service, including hospital service, on the basis of contracts with carriers for payment in advance or periodic charges. In both instances, however, the Rockefeller plan appears to rely on the removal of legal and technical barriers rather than the offer of positive inducements to form such corporations.

I suppose most of us agree that to the extent the health insurance system can use its buying power to improve the delivery system, it should do so. Perhaps the only area where doubts arise concerns the desirability of using the insurance reimbursement system to control the proliferation of facilities. Some proposals, such as the Kennedy bill, suggest that reimbursement of capital expansions or depreciation allowances should occur only if the planned expansion is certified by a state or local planning agency as being necessary or of a high order of priority. But it may be better to exclude capital costs entirely from the health insurance reimbursement formulas. Separate provision would lend itself more readily to implementing overall planning of resources, local or national. Instead of the health insurance administrator negotiating hospital by hospital to determine whether new capital additions are justifiable, needed resources would be allocated by a separate agency making allocations as indicated by the determined needs of the community or region.

But aside from this, the vital question is in what ways the health insurance plans can influence delivery systems. It is clear that great reliance is placed on "financial and other incentives." Reimbursement formulas and grants such as those proposed in the Kennedy, Javits, and Griffiths bills could increase the financial attractiveness of prepaid group practice, though it is by no means certain that the main hindrance to this form of organization is financial. But the main problem today is surely one of assuring adequate and appropriate linkages between the various types and levels of service and between primary physician care, secondary care based on community hospitals, the super specialist care of the medical center, and the supportive health services of the community.

How is this to be brought about and to whom are the incentives to be addressed? Even the Griffiths bill, which aims to assure continuity of professional treatment on the one hand and institutional care on the other, still appears to do nothing to insure that the two hands will meet; and it is doubtful how far groups of physicians will be capable of arranging for the whole gamut of professional services. Nor is it clear how enforceable is the Kennedy requirement that institutions and individual providers of care must establish working relationships with others.

Something can be done about linkages by standard setting. Thus it can be provided that any participating physician must have a hospital affiliation. But what if the hospitals refuse to accept him? Both the

Griffiths and the Kennedy bills provide that any participating hospital must not refuse affiliation for any reason other than lack of professional competence. But how can the hospitals be induced or forced to take action to raise the levels of competence of the physicians practicing in their catchment areas? How can they be induced or forced to assume some leadership in developing the community health services or to align themselves with prepaid group practice units? And if not the hospitals, what agencies or groups of people would seem to offer leadership potential?

All current health insurance proposals appear to concentrate mainly on physicians' services, broadly interpreted, and on institutional providers. But what about what might be termed the health infrastructure? By that I mean the supportive community health services on the one hand and on the other the underpinning services and procedures needed by large numbers of providers and patients and which can most effectively be provided on a large scale. I am thinking of centralized data bank and retrieval systems, multiphasic screening facilities, a comprehensive transportation system, or certain types of laboratory services. How are these to be brought into being? Should provision of such facilities be the responsibility of the health insurance system or should they be provided otherwise? And where should responsibility for assuring an adequate volume and appropriate types and distribution of medical manpower be placed?

Sooner or later, too, a decision will have to be made about the compatibility of a fee-for-service basis of professional remuneration and a system that assures comprehensive and continuous care. The AMA, the insurance companies, and Governor Rockefeller appear not to question the fee-for-service principle and propose no changes in the status quo. The Kennedy and Griffiths bills evidently regard fee-for-service as a barrier to the development of a desirable system. Griffiths proposes from the first the reimbursement of groups of providers serving defined populations through a capitation system based on a national capitation rate modified by local adjustments. The Kennedy bill encourages capitation and sometimes salary payment, but permits continuation of fee-for-service for independent providers. However, in the event of a shortage of funds, only those paid on a fee-for-service basis would suffer reductions in reimbursement.

All proposals make obeisance to the principle of free choice on the part of the patient. To the AMA and the insurance industry, this seems to mean free choice of individual physician, specialist, hospital, or insurance company. Yet increasingly today it is recognized that what is needed is free choice between systems. Now a system, as I understand it, is an articulated structure, an entity in which the various essential and functionally related components are appropriately linked. Hospital-based or connected prepaid group practice is an example of such a system. But do we have any others? If not, and the alternative is to allow free choice to select any provider, personal or institutional, to render the basic services guaranteed, does this not commit us to a reimbursement system on an item-by-item basis and to a perpetuation of fragmentation and lack of continuity?

In any event, if we really mean a choice between systems, we must ask ourselves how many systems we need in any given community, state, or region? Can we afford unlimited proliferation of competing health delivery systems any more than we can afford unlimited proliferation of facilities and costly equipment? And who is to determine how many are needed? Should this, too, be the responsi-bility, as appears to be envisaged in the Javits bill, of our emerging health planning agencies, which have hitherto concentrated mainly on planning for facilities and supply of personnel? The Kennedy bill specifically gives the health security board the power to require providers to expand, modify, or curtail offered services.

Given what would seem to be the obvious advantages of prepaid group health systems to the consumer and patient, in most respects to the practitioner, and to society at large in terms of economy, does one not have to ask why this system has not been able to enlist a more powerful constituency? Some of the reasons are clear: legal barriers in some states, opposition of organized medicine enforced by sanctions such as refusal of hospital affiliation to participating physicians, inability of group health organizations to own and control their own hospitals, problems of covering setting-up costs, difficulty of offering salaries competitive with private practice, a medical education system that builds in the emerging professional the image of the solo practitioner as the ideal to emulate and neglects the teaching of community medicine, and the lack of effective consumer education.

Probably all these have played a role, and to the extent they have we have some clues as to the steps, financial and otherwise, that have to be taken. But we also must ask why the public, which in the end always seems to get what it is really determined to have, has allowed these barriers to persist. Are there perhaps some features of current plans that repel or at least are not attractive to those who use or might use the services and to the participating professionals? Are there some obstacles to the expansion of prepaid group practice that lie within the control of the movement itself? Do they, for example, make adequate provision for a role for the consumer?

172

# The Role of the Consumer

The various health insurance plans differ considerably in the role they allot to the consumer. The AMA appears to see little place for consumer involvement. The proposal does indeed provide for a national health insurance advisory committee of nine persons but gives no specification as to the characteristics of the seven non-ex-officio members. The stress laid on developing programs to assure quality and effective utilization "through measures which provide for participation of carriers and providers" clearly reflects the AMA view, as stated by Roth[1]: "it is generally agreed by all authorities in the field that any adjudication in respect to the quality, quantity, or price tags for medical service must be made by the process of peer review. Perhaps the outstanding single advantage of our plan is that the providers of service—the only ones with the capacity to pass judgment on its equity—are maximally motivated to accept responsibility for the success of its operation." In such a philosophy there is little place for the consumer.

The Aetna proposal also includes a national advisory committee of nine persons, mainly experts but including a consumer representative. However, the plan assumes the formation of local comprehensive health planning agencies in which consumers would presumably be represented and provides that proposed institutional budgets and charges should be reviewed by a body composed of consumers, insurers, and health-care institutions.

The Rockefeller bill envisages considerable consumer involvement. The program is to be administered by a state health insurance corporation of 12 trustees, at least three of whom are to represent consumers or purchasers of health services and are to receive a salary. This body will appoint nine regional councils similarly composed. The plan also provides for public hearings on proposed premium rates and specifies that 75% of the directors of any hospital or health service corporation and 60% of the directors of a medical expense indemnity corporation must be representatives of broad segments of the subscribers covered by the contracts and other persons qualified to act in the public interest.

More explicit provision for the consumer is made by the Kennedy, Griffiths, and Javits bills. The Kennedy bill provides for a national health security advisory council of 21 members, of which a majority are to be consumers, and similarly constituted councils are envisaged at the regional and subregional levels. These bodies, which are to be assisted by technicians and secretarial staffs, are to report on all aspects of the program. The report of the national council must be submitted to the Congress by the Secretary of Health, Education and Welfare, together with a statement of his reasons for any disagreement with its recommendations. In addition, comprehensive health service organizations are required to consult periodically with enrollees.

The Griffiths plan would be administered by a 10-member national health insurance board with two members representing management and labor. There would also be an advisory health benefits council of 21 members who are "familiar with the need for personal health services in urban and rural areas as well as among the working population, the poor, the aged, children, and various minority groups." At the regional level there are to be regional consumers advisory committees of 12 to 14 persons—representatives of minority groups, the poor, the aged, labor, farmers, and consumer cooperatives—who are to be given their own professional staffs. The Griffiths and Javits bills appear to be the only ones that provide machinery for dealing with the complaints and grievances of patients or would-be patients.

The Javits bill specifies that the proposed comprehensive health service organizations must consult periodically with representatives of the membership and provide for user representation on their governing boards. In administering the loans and grants programs, the Secretary of Health, Education and Welfare must enlist consumer and community involvement in the planning, development, and operation and insure "prompt response to local initiative." And in carrying out his mandate to develop new methods of compensation, the secretary is required to consult with state and local representatives of consumers and, where none exist, to encourage and assist their establishment. In addition, he must hold hearings to obtain the views of users of the health services.

Everyone today, with the possible exception of the AMA, is talking about consumer participation and involvement. But there is a lack of agreement about what aspects of a health services program lend themselves to consumer participation, about the form that participation should take, the levels of government at which different types of consumer involvement would be most effective, and about the types of persons who can represent the interests of the consumer.

It seems clear that the consumer has many roles, and the way these can be best performed (through the ballot box, the appointment of consumer-conscious administrators, representation on governing or advisory bodies, through public hearings or organized local community councils, and the like) will vary with the different types of consumer interest in the program. As the ultimate footer of the national bill, the consumer is interested in overall costs, efficiency and economy of operation, and financial accountability. As a member of a nation seeking to make a reality of the right to needed health services, he is concerned with overall policy and its administrative implementation; that is, with performance accountability. As a member of a local community, he is interested in the appropriateness of the delivery system to the special circumstances of his area. As an individual recipient of service, he needs some way of venting his dissatisfaction with the quality or adequacy of the service he receives.

The phrases "involvement or participation of consumers at appropriate points" and "appropriate representation of consumer interests" occur in the literature with maddening frequency and a baffling lack of specificity. Identification of the different types of consumer interests and discovery of effective devices for making the consumer's voice heard and influential are major pieces of unfinished business in the development of health insurance plans.

It is evident that there will soon be major extensions of something called health insurance. The question is not "whether" but "what kind." In 1965 those of us who were concerned with the health services were caught napping. Next time we shall have no such excuse, and we have now experienced the unhappy results of our lack of preparedness. It is now generally recognized that the problem is much broader than the mere removal of the financial barrier. Study and comparison of the provisions of the various bills now before Congress, only the major features of which I have here been able to touch upon, should reveal the issues and alternatives. It should help to sharpen our thinking on two essential points; namely, the characteristics of an efficient and socially acceptable health services delivery system and the nature of the organizational structures, financial arrangements, and administrative systems most likely to bring it into effect.

## Notes

1. Roth RB: Statement on behalf of the American Medical Association. Hearings on Social Security and Welfare Proposals before the Committee on Ways and Means, House of Representatives, 91st Cong, 1st Sess. US Government Printing Office, Washington, DC, November 3-6, 1969, 1419-1457, and *Ibid:* Medicredit: A national health services financing proposal. Paper prepared for discussion at the National Health Forum, Washington, DC, February 23-25, 1970. Mimeographed.

2. Pettengill D: Statement on behalf of Aetna Life and Casualty. Hearings on Social Security and Welfare Proposals before the Committee on Ways and Means, House of Representatives, 91st Cong, 1st Sess. US Government Printing Office, Washington, DC, November 3-6, 1969, 1824-1836.

3. State of New York: Health insurance bill. Albany, 1970.

4. National Governors' Conference: System of universal health insurance. Colorado Springs, Colo., August 31-September 3, 1969.

5. US House of Representatives: Bill to provide a program of national health insurance and for other purposes. HR 15779. 91st Cong, 2d Sess. US Government

Printing Office, Washington, DC, February 9, 1970.

6. US Senate: The Health Security Act. S 4297, 91st Cong, 2d Sess. US Government Printing Office, Washington, DC, August 27, 1970. In 1971 the Griffiths and Kennedy bills were combined and introduced as HR 22 and S 3.

7. US House of Representatives: A bill to provide a program of national health insurance and for other purposes. HR 24. 91st Cong, 1st Sess. US Government Printing Office, Washington, DC, January 3, 1969.

8. US House of Representatives: A bill to provide for medical and hospital care through a system of voluntary health insurance. HR 9835. 91st Cong, 1st Sess. US Government Printing Office, Washington, DC, April 1, 1969.

9. US Senate: A bill to provide for medical and hospital care through a system of voluntary health insurance. S 2705. 91st Cong, 1st Sess. US Government Printing Office, Washington, DC, July 28, 1969.

10. US Senate: A bill concerning Medicare benefits, extension and improvement. S 3711. 91st Cong, 1d Sess. US Government Printing Office, Washington, DC, April 14, 1970.

11. President's Commission on Income Maintenance Programs: Poverty amid plenty. US Government Printing Office, Washington, DC, November 1969.

# 9

# Health Insurance: Not If, Or When, But What Kind?

In the last decade the nation's health services have been investigated as never before. Extensive hearings before the House Ways and Means Committee and the Senate Finance Committee have been accompanied by an impressive series of public and private commissions, committees of inquiry, and task forces.[1] The findings of these bodies have been depressingly monotonous. Access to needed health services is impeded by financial barriers and by an inefficient delivery system. Costs are escalating rapidly, manpower is inadequate, poorly distributed, and inefficiently utilized. Service is fragmented. The system is wasteful of resources and functions with too little regard for efficiency and economy. Current delivery arrangements appear to be devised more for the convenience of the providers than of the consumers who exercise far too little influence over what is provided and how.

There seems also to be considerable unanimity as to the objectives of reform. On at least four points there is widespread agreement. First, access to needed health services must not be impeded by financial barriers. Second, the delivery system must be one in which comprehensive and continuous health services are everywhere available under conditions that are physically convenient, comfortable, and not destructive of the dignity or self-respect of the recipient. Third, services must be provided efficiently and with due regard to economy in the use of scarce resources. Finally, the system must be accountable to those who finance it and to those who use it, and in particular must be highly responsive to the interests of consumers.

It is thus not surprising that recent months have witnessed the introduction of a large number of bills into Congress, all addressing

The Metta Bean Lecture, delivered at the University of Wisconsin, Madison, Wis., May 10, 1971, and reprinted by permission in the *American Journal of Public Health*, Vol LXI, No 11 (November 1971), 2164-2175.

themselves to the removal of the financial barrier and most of them dealing in some way or other with the delivery system. The majority of them would enact some form of "health insurance."[2]

It seems inevitable that within the next two or three years, at latest, something called a health insurance program will be enacted. The success of Medicare, even if limited, has shown that compulsory health insurance is feasible, and the rising costs of health services (including the costs of purchasing private health insurance), which now cause the middle classes and not merely the poor to wince, have stimulated a demand for extending the protections of Medicare to persons not yet 65 years old. At the same time, the high costs of even a deliberalized Medicaid program are propelling governments, both federal and state, to seek ways of financing health costs that do not fall so exclusively on the general taxpayer. We can also expect growing support for measures that aim to change the delivery system in view of the ever more vocal consumer dissatisfaction with present arrangements and the realization by large-scale financing institutions, both public and private, that the delivery system is inefficient and uneconomic and is itself contributing to the rising costs which are acutely embarrassing both groups. Thus the question that must concern us is not whether or when we shall have some kind of health insurance legislation on the books, but rather, what kind of health insurance system shall we have? For although, as I have stated, there is considerable agreement as to the ends it is desired to attain, there is much difference of opinion as to how these objectives are to be achieved.

## Removal of the Financial Barrier

The major objective of all proposals currently before the Congress is removal of financial barriers. All bills would utilize some form of insurance, a system of prepayment on the part of members of a group in return for which they are entitled to specific benefits in cash or kind in specified contingencies. But here the resemblance stops. First, some plans such as those of the AMA and in part those of the Health Insurance Association of America (HIAA) provide for voluntary insurance coverage. Others such as the Javits, Griffiths and Kennedy bills, require compulsory coverage. Only one of the three new schemes proposed by President Nixon is compulsory.[3] Second, some would cover the entire population by a single system (e.g., the Griffiths and Kennedy bills), while others, such as the AMA, the HIAA, and the Nixon plans envisage two or more systems, usually differentiated by reference to the income level of the insured.[4] Third, some provide for a sizable contribution from the federal revenues to a single national system (Griffiths, Javits, and Kennedy) while others (the HIAA proposal or the Nixon plan) provide that, in their dual systems, one program should be financed by wage and payroll taxes alone, while another should carry a government subsidy.[5] Fourth, the plans differ in the extent to which the insured are required to shoulder at least some of the costs (over and above payment of premiums or social insurance taxes). Thus some exclude certain types of health services or limit the duration of their receipt—even the Kennedy bill, the most inclusive of all, restricts dental care to children below a certain age and sets a limit to the duration of nursing home care. In addition, most plans embody deductibles, coinsurance and copayment. Here again the Kennedy bill is a notable exception.

Finally, the plans differ in that some envisage a wholly federal program whereas others, such as the insurance company proposals and those of the American Hospital Association, rely heavily on state initiative, often with partial financing and administration of the new schemes, or else by proposing continuation of Medicaid again rely on state action (e.g., the Nixon proposals and the AMA plans).

How do these policies affect attainment of the objective of removal of the financial barrier? Clearly, limited benefit coverage and sizable cost sharing through deductibles, coinsurance, and copayments will mean that for many families, especially those who are poorer, the costs of needed health services will continue to be prohibitive or ruinous. We already know that Medicare has removed only about half of the financial barriers for the aged. Limited coverage may be inevitable initially in view of shortages of resources, both personal and institutional. But this means that in evaluating the plans, special attention must be paid to what proposals are included in them for remedying these deficiencies.

The use of cost-sharing devices is generally ascribed to a desire to control overuse of the service. Since these both perpetuate the financial barrier and discourage early utilization of health services, more attention should be paid to controls other than those that bear on the patient. This is especially appropriate in such a service as health, where decisions as to the nature and extent of services to be utilized are largely in the hands of professional providers.

A program that relies solely on wage and payroll taxes for its support is likely to be a limited program in terms of both coverage and benefits, because of the impossibility (or at least the difficulty) of collecting full actuarial contributions from lower paid workers, let alone from those who are not employed.[6] Full coverage will not be achieved without a sizable contribution from the general revenues.

The experience of other countries, and indeed our own with Part B of Medicare, has shown that 100% coverage cannot be achieved by even a subsidized voluntary plan. Similarly, our past experience with public assistance medical care, with the Kerr-Mills program, and more recently with Medicaid has demonstrated beyond argument that any program relying for its implementation on state initiative and substantial, or even not so substantial, state financing will never bring about removal of the financial barrier in the nation as a whole.

Thus far we can decide for or against specific policies on what might be termed technical or experience grounds. When one has to choose between coverage systems that do or do not involve demonstrations of income inadequacy (such as the public assistance or Medicaid approach or the subsidized insurance plans as proposed by the AMA, the nonfringe benefit type of coverage of HIAA or President Nixon's Family Insurance Plan) the choice has to be made primarily on the basis of values.[7] Essentially, it is a matter of how one feels about the further extension of income tests to ever larger segments of the population, on the one hand, and on the other, how much importance one attaches to ensuring that every person, except perhaps those under the current poverty line, should contribute toward the cost of his health care.[8] One of the most crucial issues we face is whether there is any place, in a service as basic as health, for perpetuation of the income test approach, especially when we have already rejected it in another basic service— namely, elementary and high school education.

## Comprehensive and Continuous Care

Achievement of the second widely agreed on objective—that the services must be everywhere available, comprehensive, nonfragmented and furnished on a coordinated basis—raises fewer value issues but presents many more technical problems. Essentially the task is twofold: assuring the availability of resources and creating effective linkages between them.

Most of the proposals deal in one way or another with the problem of resources, though the plans are sometimes embodied in legislation separate from the health insurance bill itself. There is a remarkable measure of agreement as to what is needed. Although the need for more physicians is recognized, all proposals place considerable emphasis on the production of additional paramedical personnel and include a variety of financial incentives to encourage their training and use. Perhaps the most original, as it is the most dubious of the aids to

180

professional education, is the Nixon proposal to make grants to medical schools in proportion to the numbers they graduate. All major proposals too take note of the maldistribution of professional personnel, and here again the main instrument to bring about change is financial, although some, such as the Nixon proposals and those of the Carnegie Commission on Higher Education, would encourage the creation of health education centers in underdoctored areas and other aids to offset professional isolation of practice in certain parts of the country. Here the main question is a technical one: will these inducements prove effective or will the country in the end have to adopt some more drastic control over professional location?

Most of the plans, other than those of the AMA and HIAA, aim to do something about assurance of adequate facilities. Differences here seem to relate to two points: the extent to which capital costs should be subsidized or reimbursed as an integral part of the financing of the insurance system and the extent to which financial aid, whether in the form of reimbursement through the insurance system or through an independent health facility financing body, should require conformity with state or local planning bodies' schemes.

Orderly linkages between the different parts of the health services system (preventive and primary care, specialized service, appropriate institutional care, domiciliary and community health services) could in principle be assured by a single provider system responsible to a single authority. No such organization exists, to my knowledge, outside the communist countries. Even the British Health Service, which has nationalized the hospitals, required specialists to be attached to them, and compelled primary physicians desiring to practice under the system to accept a capitation method of payment for enrolled potential patients, has failed to fully integrate the locally run health services into the program, and the relations of the GP's, the specialists and the hospitals are not all that could be desired. In any case, it is unlikely that the British example will be followed in the near future in this country. Instead, our present policy seems to be to seek for some smaller unit of organization for patient care that would contract with government to provide the full spectrum of needed health services, both personal and institutional, for an enrolled population in return for a capitation payment. Prepaid group practice, under a variety of new names, has suddenly become fashionable and is apparently the model that is to be the answer to prayer. I say "apparently" because in all proposals and discussions of the health services of the future, one finds reference to "experimentation," "innovation," and "imaginative proposals" that are to be encouraged in every way. It would be helpful if the proponents of

181

experimentation were to be somewhat more specific about the kind of experimentation they have in mind. Is it some departure from the central concepts of group practice, namely that of a single-door entrance to all needed services and a single organization responsible for seeing that they are indeed available to its membership? Or is it experimentation within this model, e.g., with different kinds of sponsorship, different systems of remunerating the group or the individual professional providers, or different kinds of linkages between the components of the system, or different roles for the consumers?

Assuming, however, that some form of prepaid group practice, whether bearing the name of Senator Javits' "local comprehensive health service system" or Senator Kennedy's "comprehensive health service organizations" or the American Hospital Association's "health care corporations" or President Nixon's "health maintenance organization," is indeed the preferred model, how is it to be brought into being? It cannot be done by limiting participation in the publicly supported program to organizations of this kind, for they are today far too few, and it would take several years before they could offer anything like national coverage. Even so, it might be desirable to set some future date by which time fee-for-service payment of services on an item-by-item basis would no longer be acceptable under the public program.

All current health insurance plans, other than that of the AMA, contain provisions aiming to encourage the development of such care systems. They range from the somewhat optimistic reliance of the American Hospital Association on "the strong demand for these changes by those who use and finance health care," as the lever to motivate providers, through the modest proposals of the HIAA plan for the training of physicians to function in groups, to very extensive financial inducements, such as grants for planning, loans and grants for construction, financial assistance in developing management and statistical systems, underwriting the setting-up costs, and the like. Other inducements take the form of steps to remove state legislative barriers to group practice. In addition, the earlier Kennedy bill would have utilized the provider payment arrangements of the health insurance system to place professionals functioning in group systems in a preferential position as compared with those in solo or independent practice.

There is indeed a surprising uniformity about the types of inducements that are provided for in the various proposals.[9] The impact of these measures on the health service delivery system will, however, depend on (a) how effective the financial inducements prove to be in practice; (b) who will organize such groups; (c) the nature of the standards laid down for participation; (d) how far it will prove feasible to monitor such systems to ensure that quality is not sacrificed to cost-saving; and finally (e) how successfully the general public is induced to prefer this type of delivery system, a point to which so far too little attention has been paid.[10]

Of these, perhaps the most crucial is who will organize the comprehensive delivery systems? Will the initiative come from medical centers, hospitals, groups of physicians, consumer cooperatives, large-scale unions, private insurance companies, or entrepreneurs hitherto unconnected with the health industry, who, as has been the case with nursing homes since 1965, will see in the liberal subsidy or reimbursement offers a prospect of profitable investment at little risk? The danger will be that the desire rapidly to develop these organizations on a large scale may lead to uncritical acceptance of the wrong kind of sponsorship.

The favored candidates today seem to be the hospitals and the insurance companies, although most plans express the hope that groups of physicians will be motivated to action. Surprisingly little emphasis seems to be placed on consumer cooperatives or other nonprofit groups representing the consumer.

The role to be assigned to insurance companies, profit and nonprofit, differs considerably among the plans. The Kennedy bill would exclude them entirely, except for their possible initial use as administrative agents. On the other hand the AMA, the HIAA plans, and the Nixon proposals would give them a central position, since the essence of these plans is a legal compulsion on employers to provide health insurance as a fringe benefit plus a system of federal subsidies to permit everyone to purchase private health insurance.[11] Senator Javits would use them as administrative agencies as in Medicare and rely heavily on them for initiative in changing the delivery system, while his provisions for contracting out and choice of "alternative systems" would utilize private insurance companies.

Yet in a system providing for compulsory coverage and which is to operate on a service rather than an indemnity basis with delivery through forms of group practice remunerated on a capitation basis, it is increasingly difficult to see a role for private insurance institutions. Assuming compulsory insurance contributions, there is no need for any agency other than the tax collector to see that people belong to the insurance system. And only if it could be argued that the government lacks the administrative ability to monitor the program and administer the remuneration of providers, would there be a strong case for utilizing the private insurance agencies as administrative intermediaries. Actually, I believe it will be harder and harder to maintain this argument. The federal government is becoming increasingly sophisticated in its awareness of the administrative issues and, under congressional pressure, is already beginning to exercise more influence over what is done. The record of the private insurance intermediaries under Medicare is not so spectacularly good as to provide overwhelming support for their continued use. Finally, and most important, the type of delivery system envisaged by all proposals, except perhaps those of the AMA, is not a system in regard to which private insurance companies have particular expertise or extensive experience. They are familiar with the indemnity approach with its itemized reimbursement arrangements but have little more experience than government agencies with adminstration of comprehensive service plans utilizing a capitation system where proper administration involves the financing authority, on behalf of the enrolled membership, in questions of quality of service, adequacy of linkages, and the like.

In view of what one hears about the extent to which the insurance companies are losing money on their health insurance business, one may wonder why they are so eager to remain in the field, unless it is that they hope that once ensconced in the program, they will be able to exert pressure on the government to provide ever higher premium subsidies as costs rise. In fact, it is not always clear how far the various plans would allow the companies to make a profit. The Kennedy bill would prohibit profit-making in the comprehensive health service, but apparently permits it in private practice. Presumably the Nixon and HIAA plans assume that the newly compulsory fringe health benefits will be bought, as now, from profit-making insurance companies. But what about the business the companies would get as a result of the subsidized premiums of the nonemployed and the poor? Are these also to include a profit? One presumes so in view of the references in the Nixon proposals to intensive competition among insurance companies for this business.

But one may ask whether, in a system where henceforth the business done by insurance companies would be so largely dependent on government action, there is any justification for permitting profit-making in the dispensing of the funds. In any case, the use of private intermediaries operating for profit will necessitate a vast dual control system, for the government will have to monitor their performance and set standards for operation that cover more than a definition of the basic health package that is to be sold and may well extend to permitted charges and profits.

184

If, however, there is to be no profit one may wonder why, apart from a concern about job security for their present employees (an important political factor) the private companies will be eager to remain in the business. So long as the governmental program, as with Medicare, was small in relation to the coverage of private business, one could understand a willingness to act as a nonprofit-making intermediary as a good-will activity and an entering wedge for other profitable business. But the situation would be different with a national compulsory or governmentally subsidized health insurance system with extensive coverage, accompanied by governmental regulation of the insurance industry.

## Efficiency and the Economical Use of Resources

All current health insurance proposals contain provisions directed toward the objective of efficiency and the economical use of resources. Several major approaches can be identified. First, some would utilize the arrangements for reimbursement of providers. These include rather generally the substitution of a predetermined budget for the present end-of-year, essentially cost-plus basis of remuneration, building in financial inducements to efficiency by permitting retention of all or part of any savings they are able to make. Proposals for encouraging economical operation through modifications of the reimbursement arrangements, however, seem to be less common and specific for professional noninstitutional-based service providers. The plans variously propose adoption of fee schedules or value scales, or limitation of fees by reference to changes in the cost-of-living index or some other national index, or setting a limit by reference to some specified percentile of prevailing charges at some designated date. The effectiveness of thsee controls is, however, yet to be demonstrated, and most plans require the federal government to undertake or promote research into reimbursement or remuneration systems.

A second approach, as already indicated, is the encouragement of delivery systems that are believed to be more efficient. Indeed, in some plans (the Nixon proposals), the presumed cost savings seem to be the main attraction of the new system. While the capitation-financed group practice system is undoubtedly capable of providing better service to patients, there appears to be still some question as to the financial savings it makes possible, when account is taken of quality differentials (e.g., is utilization of hospitalization limited solely by medical considerations?) or of the extent to which the membership utilizes and pays for services outside the system.

A third approach is the overt discouragement of overuse or improper

185

use of resources. Overuse of existing services is, as already mentioned, supposedly controlled by the use of cost-sharing devices and by requiring the appointment of utilization committees and peer review of the appropriateness of services rendered. But here again, peer review is likely to be most effective in the case of institutionally based services, and even here the reports to date have not been too encouraging. Little serious effort seems as yet to have been made to monitor, let alone control, the efficient and economical functioning of the independent or solo practitioner.[12]

Almost all plans make some effort to control the volume of resources, both personal and facilities, devoted to the health service industry. The most usual control on investment in facilities seems to be the requirement for conformity with state or local health plans as a condition for receipt of public loans or grants. Only the Nixon plan appears to place little reliance on such planning. Economic use of manpower is to be fostered in almost all plans by financial aid for the training of paraprofessionals (the Nixon and Kennedy proposals contain a variety of incentives for the development of such personnel) and in addition, the Kennedy bill would encourage the utilization of local residents.

Finally, all plans give at least lip service to the encouragement of preventive action as a method of keeping down costs. These efforts take the form of removal of present discouragements to prevention (such as the exclusion of preventive checkups from reimbursable services) and adoption of a system of remuneration, namely capitation, that is believed to make preventive care profitable, by encouragement of health education of the population and finally by stimulus of research into prevention of potentially controllable causes of ill health (e.g., President Nixon's proposals for research into accidents, cancer, and sickle-cell anemia).

These efforts to assure economical and efficient operation of the health services raise a number of questions. The most obvious is, of course, will they work? Here only experience will show, although at least in regard to the last of them, encouragement of prevention, it seems likely that additional investments in income adequacy, decent housing, adequate nutrition, and environmental purification would be more effective promoters of health than efforts directed to the eradication of certain diseases. Almost all of the proposals rely on financial inducements or incentives: little is said about direct controls over both overuse and the opposite danger that emphasis on economy may lead to diminution of quality. At least one large public purchaser of care, New York City, has found it essential to develop a service auditing system with penalties in the form of refusal to reimburse those found guilty of overservicing, grossly deficient quality, or fraud.[13]

## Accountability and Responsiveness to Consumers

Accountability has two facets: financial and performance. Hitherto attention has mainly focused on the former. Even here, as we have seen, it cannot as yet be claimed that full success has been achieved, especially in regard to noninstitutionally connected professional providers. Performance accountability necessitates a definition of the services to be provided in terms of both quantity and quality. From this point of view the proposed shift to predetermined budgeting should be helpful, for it will require specification of the type, level, and scope of services to be provided by the contractor. Much needs to be done, however, to develop techniques and tools of surveillance. One thing is clear, namely that accountability of both types will be more readily achieved the fewer the independent providers and the less fragmented the delivery system.

From the national point of view a major lack is the absence of some overall federal agency charged with the task of specifying national goals, defining standards of performance and regularly reporting to the country on progress or its absence. A number of the plans recognize this: differences turn mainly on the locus of such a body, whether it should be similar in status and location to the Council of Economic Advisors or should be the Health Security Board itself, or an advisory body attached to the federal administration or to the Secretary of Health, Education and Welfare.

Performance accountability is also the objective of the many proposals found in current bills for consumer representation; indeed, only the President's message and the AMA appear to envisage no special role for the consumer. Here is an area where much experimentation seems called for; experimentation in regard to the structural arrangements for consumer influence, the types of people who should serve on what kinds of consumer representative bodies and the like. This is an area where values are less influential in decision-making than are technical considerations, for at least lip service is now given to the view that the consumer should exert influence over the health services and their system of delivery.

## Techniques and Values

The decisions that will have to be made involve both technical questions (e.g., will such and such an incentive work? How can consumer interest best be organized?) on the one hand and on the other, value judgments. In regard to the latter, I believe that the task of devising an acceptable system will be less difficult if we can avoid being mesmerized by impressive-sounding big words. For too long, the AMA was able to petrify thinking about basic changes in the organization and financing of the health services by applying the pejorative term "socialized medicine" to every proposed change. Not enough people asked, "What exactly is socialized medicine and what's wrong with it anyway?" The exorcising power of this particular incantation seems now to be less effective. But there are other mesmerizing words of which we must beware.

One of these is "pluralism," which we are told, does now and must always characterize our health services and which is contrasted with the dirty word "monolithic." Exactly what a pluralistic system means is not easy to say. To President Nixon it is a system "which creates many effective centers of responsibility—both public and private—rather than one that concentrates authority in a single governmental source."[14] But isn't this diffused responsibility exactly what is wrong with the present system? Do we not have to insist that there are some aspects of the health industry where we cannot have multiple responsibility? Even Mr. Nixon proposes to concentrate in the federal government responsibility for determining the content of the minimum package of benefits that employers must provide and hints that the federal government may take further steps to regulate private insurance. Nor would he share with the states the decision as to the legality of group practice. In fact, of course, none of the current health insurance proposals is monolithic in the sense that *all* policy decisions *and their implementation* are concentrated in the hands of the federal government. Our problem is precisely that of determining which aspects of the health services system lend themselves to multiple and which necessitate a single center of responsibility. In considering this question it is helpful to distinguish between the responsibility to see that something is done and the actual doing of it.

It does not help to talk about pluralism in vague terms. Indeed, one is tempted to think that the emphasis on this concept in some quarters is a facade to cover a plea for continued involvement of private insurance companies in whatever arrangement is finally adopted and for perpetuation of the freedom of providers, especially hospitals and physicians, to continue to function as they have always done in the past.

"Freedom" is another magic word of which we must beware. We are told that freedom must always be preserved. But once again we must insist on being specific and ask, "freedom to do what and for whom?" In the context of the health services, "freedom" would seem to have several connotations. The most usually cited freedom is the freedom of the patient to choose his doctor. Yet we have already seen that technological developments have largely limited this freedom today to the choice of the primary physician or specialist, even for the most affluent and well-informed, serving as the point of entry to whatever series of procedures is indicated. Certainly, for the majority this freedom is further restricted by the nonavailability of professional personnel or by financial considerations, and for the poor it hardly exists at all. In this respect, all plans that would eliminate or lower the financial barrier are enlarging the freedom of choice of most patients. None would seem to place additional restrictions on this freedom, although membership in a group practice organization or HMO would presumably involve some limit on the frequency with which this freedom can be exercised, since the shift of patients from one system to another complicates the financial and other arrangements.

Freedom for the health services consumer can also imply the right to decide what kind of system he will utilize. The present choice would seem to be (a) between some form of prepaid group practice, where available, and purchase from independent providers on an item-by-item basis, and (b) between competing group providers or competing independent providers. Enticing as this high degree of freedom may sound, one may nevertheless ask how far society can afford to grant or encourage it in the basic health services system. Given the importance of conserving resources and assuming that the group practice model is indeed a more efficient system for rendering care, should social policy not seek deliberately to narrow the choice of system?

It is not only the consumers whose absolute freedom of choice may have to be restricted. Providers are also affected. President Nixon has stated that among the strengths of the existing system "is the diversity of our system and the range of choice it therefore provides for *doctors* [my italics] and patients alike." The doctor's choices would seem to relate to (a) under what kind of system he will practice; (b) where geographically he will practice; and (c) what kind of medicine (clinical, research, specialist or family physician, etc.) he will practice. I have already suggested that the first of these freedoms may have to be limited as the pressure for economy of operation becomes more intense. The undesirable consequences of the second unrestricted freedom are all too apparent, while the third becomes ever harder to justify as society assumes ever larger financial responsibility for

189

professional education. Our problem is how to limit these freedoms in an acceptable manner. To the extent that current proposals deal with these problems, they do so in a nice, polite way through the use of financial incentives. Only experience will show whether we shall have to supplement these incentives by more direct controls.

Freedom to invest resources in health service facilities is increasingly coming into question and we can expect a variety of efforts to limit it by putting teeth into state and local planning through the power to withhold financial aid for disapproved construction. Finally, the problem of freedom arises in a new form as efforts are made to encourage the growth of the prepaid comprehensive group practice type of delivery system. Is anyone or any group to be free to go into the business? On the one hand, one can ask how much cutthroat competition the consumer can productively cope with—how much fine print will he be able to read and understand? On the other hand, recognizing that the organization and operation of these supply systems involve a sizable investment of capital and above all of scarce human organizing resources, we must ask how many of them make sense in any given area.

Development of the health services in the next few years will be both exciting and determinative. It is of vital importance that we never lose sight of our major objectives. Overcoming the financial barrier is indeed crucial, but of equal importance is the development of a delivery system that serves people better, uses resources economically and is accountable to those who pay for it and those who use it. These are the tests we must apply to all current proposals.

## Notes

1. Among the most important have been the Joint Commission on Mental Illness and Health (1961), the National Advisory Commission on Health Manpower (1967), the National Commission on Health Facilities (1968), the Secretary's Advisory Committee on Hospital Effectiveness (the Barr Report, 1968), the Report of the Task Force on Medicaid and Related Programs (the McNerney Report, 1970), and Mayor Lindsay's Commission on the Delivery of Personal Health Services (ND) and private studies such as the American Medical Association's Report on the Graduate Education of Physicians (the Millis Report, 1967), the Carnegie Foundation Report on Higher Education and the Nation's Health (1970), and the American Hospital Association's 1970 Report of a Special Committee on the Provision of Health Services (the so-called Ameriplan). In 1971 an advisory group of businessmen forming Governor Rockefeller's Social Services Steering Committee issued a report on Health and Hospital Services and Costs (the Wilson Report).

2. See for example the proposals of the AMA originally put forward in 1969 and embodied in HR 4960 in 1971, and those of the Health Insurance Association of America originally formulated by the Aetna Insurance Company and embodied in HR 4349 in 1971, and the bills introduced by Senator Javits (S 3711 of 1970 and S 836 of 1971), Senator Kennedy (S 3 of 1971 embodying a merger of the Kennedy 1970 bill and that of Congressman Griffith's 1970 bill, HR 15779),

Senator Bennett, whose bill S 1623 of 1971 embodied the Nixon proposals (House version of the bill introduced by Congressman Byrnes as HR 7741) and Senator Long (S 1376 of 1971).

3. Even here there is compulsion only on the employer to set up a health insurance fringe benefit plan. But there is no compulsion on workers to join and pay their share of the premium.

4. Indeed, the Nixon national health strategy envisages seven public systems: (a) national health insurance for employed persons and their families supported by wage and payroll taxes; (b) family health insurance, subsidized by the federal government for poor families with children headed by employed and unemployed persons with family incomes of under $5,000; (c) a system of special insurance pools in each state which would offer insurance at reasonable group rates to people who do not qualify for other programs; (d) Medicaid for the aged poor, blind and disabled and foster children; (e) Medicare, as now, for the aged; (f) continuation of existing federal programs for members of the armed forces (and presumably veterans) and civilian federal employees; and (g) continuation of the state and locally financied means-test medical care for persons excluded from, or inadequately covered by, any of the above systems.

5. The proposals of the American Hospital Association (Ameriplan) differ from the general pattern in providing for a threefold program of benefits; the first, health maintenance and catastrophic insurance, would be financed by social security taxes but the federal government would subsidize premiums for the poor and near-poor. The second, membership of which is a condition of coverage by the first program, provides a system of standard health benefits, and would be financed by voluntary and private purchase of insurance, although the federal government would again subsidize premiums for the poor and near-poor. The third part consists of a system of supplementary benefits to cover the gap between the benefits available under the two other programs and would be voluntary and financed by purchase of private insurance with no public subsidy. American Hospital Association Report of a Special Committee on Provision of Health Services, 1970, 8-10.

6. Many employers, too, especially small firms or direct consumers of labor services such as employers of domestic workers, would find it difficult to pay a heavy share of the actuarial premium. In recognition of this fact, Congressman Byrnes, in introducing the Nixon bill, took the unusual step of adding an amendment of his own to provide subsidies to employers.

7. Except that technical and administrative considerations might prove decisive in those plans which vary the amount of the public subsidy with the size of the insured person's income (in contrast, for instance, to the policy in Part B of Medicare where the subsidy is the same for everyone).

8. Cf the American Hospital Association, "One of the basic precepts of Ameriplan would be that within reasonable limits, those who are able to pay for their care should do so" (p 10).

9. For a more detailed account of the various proposals see above, Chapter 8.

10. For an account of the difficulties to be encountered, see Marketing of new group practice plan in Columbia described, *Group Health and Welfare News,* June 7, 1970.

11. The American Hospital Association would utilize private insurance "wherever possible."

12. Except perhaps in regard to drugs and appliances where some plans would utilize approved lists of items that could be freely prescribed.

13. See testimony of Dr. Lowell E. Bellin, First Deputy Commissioner of the Department of Health, New York City, before the Senate Subcommittee on Medicare-Medicaid, June 2, 1970, 511-538.

14. Message from the President of the United States relative to Building a National Health Strategy, 1971, p 4. See also the American Hospital Association, "In order to maximize innovation and preserve the benefits of multiple choice, the system must consist of a multiplicity of organizations with varied types of ownership and organizational forms," American Hospital Association, op cit, 5.

# 10 Health Service Policies: In Evolution Toward What?

The people need a substantially larger volume of scientific medical service than they now receive. . . . There is need for a geographical distribution of practitioners and agencies which more closely approximates the medical requirements of the people. . . . There needs to be better control over the quality of medical service. . . . The prevailing methods of purchasing medical care have unsatisfactory consequences. They lead to unwise and undirected expenditures, to unequal and unpredictable financial burdens for the individual and the family, to neglect of health and of illness, to inadequate expenditures for medical care and often to unequal remuneration of practitioners. There needs to be some plan whereby the unequal and sometimes crushing burden of medical expenses can be distributed. . . . Physical facilities are duplicated between the hospitals and the offices of practitioners and are insufficiently utilized in both. . . . Misdirected expenditures, competition and excessive specialization among practitioners and the absence of community planning and of integration of services and facilities contribute to extensive waste.[1]

It is depressing to realize that these words were not written in 1972 but were the conclusions of a distinguished and representative committee forty years ago, after a five-year study of America's health system. Indeed, as one rereads the report of the Committee on the Costs

Parts of this chapter were originally published in *American Behavioral Scientist*, May 1971, under the title "The Nation's Insurance and Health Services Policies: In Evolution Towards What?" and are reproduced by agreement with Sage Publications, Inc.

of Medical Care (CCMC) today, it is difficult not to believe that it is yet one more of the many reports emanating from the numerous committees, commissions, and task forces that have subjected America's health system to critical scrutiny in the last decade.[2]

## The Past

The intervening years have indeed seen many changes, but too many of them have served merely to intensify the problems to which the CCMC drew attention. There have been tremendous advances in the science and technology of medicine but these have led to a further growth of specialization of both practitioners and agencies which in turn has fostered fragmentation of care. Geographical maldistribution of personnel and facilities is, if anything, worse than it was in 1932, due to the movement of the middle classes out of the central cities and the influx of the impoverished, while rural and sparsely populated areas have failed to attract practitioners. The costs of medical care have become even more onerous, due to the broadened spectrum of care that now characterizes what is regarded as good modern medical practice. Additionally, the prices of both institutional and professional services have risen sharply, a trend that has been especially marked since the infusion of additional funds for the purchase of care, after the Social Security Amendments of 1965. The growing affluence of the country in the last 40 years has not offset these rising costs. A disturbingly large proportion of the population has failed to share in this affluence, and the magnitude of the costs has been so great that they constitute a serious problem even for the middle classes. Waste of resources, which also adds to costs, is if anything a more serious problem than it was in 1932 due both to the vastly greater volume of expensive equipment that is called for and the desire of prestige-seeking hospitals to be as up-to-date and "advanced" as their competitors and to the ever longer and more expensive training of physicians which increases the waste that occurs when such personnel perform functions that could well be carried out by less expensively trained personnel.

The Committee saw health insurance as the main answer to the financial problem, although only voluntary insurance was recommended by the majority. In this area there has indeed been a vast change, and the growth of private health insurance is one of the more striking developments since 1932, but it has failed to solve the financial problems of families needing medical care.[3] Less change has taken place in regard to the CCMC recommendation that consumers, on the basis of per capita payments, should arrange with an organized group of medical practitioners to furnish them with complete or virtually complete medical service. Prepaid group practice has hitherto grown but slowly and has had an uphill fight to reach even its present modest coverage.[4]

Perhaps the most impressive and undoubtedly the most influential of all trends in the last forty years has been the changed attitudes and demands of the consumers of the health services. A better educated and more sophisticated population has lost much of its earlier veneration of the medical profession and increasingly regards the health services system as an industry which, like other industries, must be accountable and responsive to the consumer. Dissatisfaction with a system that has hitherto been run primarily in the interests and for the convenience of the providers has taken the form of demands for a greater role for the consumer, more attention to the availability of services, and a delivery system that is convenient for the users, nonfragmented, and provided under conditions that do not demean human dignity. The dual system of medical care, one for the poor and one for the rest of the population, is also increasingly under attack. There is now a widespread tendency to regard access to needed health services as a right of all citizens.

This changed attitude has led, notably, to a greater use of government as an instrument for bringing about reform. The CCMC saw but a minimum role for involvement of government.[5] Over this period, and notably during the 1960's, governments (mainly the federal government) have assumed responsibilities for supporting increases in the supply of medical facilities and personnel, for operating programs directed toward meeting the costs of personal health services, for supporting extensive medical research, and for encouraging, through financial aid, state and local and regional planning of health services. These are additional to earlier and continuing responsibilities for "public health" in the traditional sense, for licensing of institutions and personnel and for the direct provision of health services for such groups as the tubercular, the mentally ill, the armed services, veterans and Indians.[6] One measure of the change is financial. In 1928-1929, when total national health expenditures amounted to $3.589 billion (3.6% of gross national product), the public sector accounted for only $477 million, or 13.3% of the total. By fiscal 1970-1971, the total had swollen to $175.0 billion (7.4% of gross national product); $28.5 billion, or 37.9%, was funded by government. The proportion of personal health expenditures paid for by government rose in the same period from 8.9 to 35.8%.[7]

# The Present

Of the expanded governmental activities, the programs initiated in 1965—Medicare and Medicaid—were undoubtedly the most far-reaching in their repercussions. Medicare introduced the use of compulsory health insurance, albeit only for the aged, but adoption of the policy was the more significant because of the heavy opposition of the medical profession and the long duration of the struggle to secure even this modest step. The importance of Medicare lay in its demonstration that federal compulsory health insurance was indeed workable and the popularity of the measure has already led to demands, some of which have been embodied in legislative proposals, for the extension of coverage to other age groups. Medicaid established the policy that no person should be prevented by financial obstacles from obtaining needed medical care. Although full attainment of the goal was not immediately envisaged, the act specified that by 1975 full coverage of the population and a full range of services should be available or concretely planned for and well on the way. Nor was the public assurance of care to be limited to those who were technically classified as poor, and thus eligible for public assistance: the act covered also the so-called "medically indigent."

Yet in the seven years after Medicare and Medicaid were enacted, health planners had already learned some lessons from bitter experience. First, it became evident that a program that operates on the principle of reimbursement for some types or forms of medical services has many grave disadvantages, especially when, as is the case with Medicare, it is accompanied by deductibles, coinsurance, and copayment requirements. It fails to remove, or even largely reduce, the financial barrier and the insured person is left with a sizable bill to pay. It has been estimated that Medicare meets rather less than half the medical care costs of the aged. The item-by-item approach also fosters fragmentation of service and encourages the use of those services for which there is whole or partial reimbursement.

Second, both Medicare and Medicaid have highlighted the crucial importance of the methods of remunerating providers. The unfortunate decision to remunerate institutional providers on what is essentially a cost-plus basis, together with a liberal interpretation of the items to be included in "reasonable costs," have encouraged neither efficiency nor economy. Costs have escalated sharply and the shortcomings of the system have been documented by a long series of committees of inquiry and Congressional hearings.[8] The years 1970 and 1971 saw a proliferation of legislative proposals for cost containment, notably those embodied in 1971 in Title II of H.R. 1 (the controversial Welfare Reform Bill) and in almost all the Health Insurance Bills.

These proposals have been primarily directed at institutional providers, but the prevailing policies governing the remuneration of individual professional providers have been equally unsatisfactory and have also encouraged cost escalation. Presumably to placate the medical profession, reimbursement has taken the form of payment of "reasonable charges," which reflect those customarily charged by the provider and those prevailing in his locality.[9]

Within the guidelines promulgated by the Social Security Administration, control over the reasonableness of costs and charges is mainly in the hands of fiscal intermediaries, private profit and nonprofit insurance companies, another concession to medical and insurance interests, although perhaps understandable in view of the enormous administrative task that initially faced the Social Security Administration. Hitherto, the record of the intermediaries in ensuring economy and restraint in price-fixing has not been impressive.[10] Nor would it seem reasonable to expect that agencies which compete for the non-Medicare business of institutions and professional providers would be eager to build up a reputation for rigorous scrutiny of charges and keeping costs to a minimum.

Third, Medicaid experience has demonstrated the limitations of reliance on state action, even with significant federal aid, to remove the financial barrier and assure access to needed health services. As of June, 1971, only 28 states had extended Medicaid coverage to the medically needy, and many states, as they have faced the costliness of the program, have reacted by cutting the services offered, and excluding some of the groups previously eligible. It has become evident that the economic position of many states precludes expenditures of the magnitude that full implementation of Medicaid would require, while others which could meet these costs from current state and local revenues are unwilling to do so because they have other priorities, including a desire to keep taxes low. The federal government, far from giving additional financial help to the states, has also reacted to rising costs by mandating a low income eligibility level and permitting states to narrow the scope of services.[11]

Fourth, Medicaid has demonstrated the undesirability of lodging administration of a health service at both federal and state levels in the hands of welfare rather than health departments. Identification of the program with the welfare system, at a time when welfare is everywhere under attack and vastly unpopular, not only serves to discourage some eligible persons from applying but probably also tends to limit appropriations, for legislatures have traditionally been more favorable to health than to welfare programs. Nor have the welfare departments been notable for a concern about quality of care. But most importantly, if there is ultimately to be an effective national health system, it will need to be supported by strong health departments—and Medicaid missed the opportunity to strengthen them (as the welfare departments were strengthened by the public assistance Titles of the Social Security Act) by giving them specific responsibilities, federal financial aid, and the imposition of federal standards.

Fifth, the 1965 policy involved the simultaneous operation of a nonmeans-test program (Medicare) and a large means-test program (Medicaid), and this has served to perpetuate a two-class health services system. The range of benefits available to the Medicaid population is much narrower, in most states, than that available to Medicare beneficiaries; physicians in some cases have refused to serve Medicaid patients (the Hippocratic oath notwithstanding) because they are dissatisfied with state reimbursement levels or procedures, and as Medicaid eligibility and covered services have been restricted, more and more poorer citizens are forced to seek care from overtaxed municipal public hospitals and clinics.

Sixth, it has become painfully evident that programs such as Medicare and Medicaid, which are directed solely to removal of the financial barrier, have a minimal effect on the nature of the admittedly unsatisfactory delivery system and on the enhancement of quality. Indeed, since their major impact is the infusion of additional funds, they may even have served to reduce consumer pressure on providers for change.

This noninvolvement of government with the delivery system and the organization and administration of health services was deliberate and explicitly stated in the preamble to Title XVIII of the 1965 amendments. But the rising expenditures under both Medicare and Medicaid and the realization that the delivery system itself is in part responsible for high costs have shown the untenability of this renunciation. More and more legislative proposals now envisage a considerable federal involvement in the health services delivery system.

Finally, experience with Medicare and Medicaid has shown that achievement of the objective of assurance of access, regardless of income levels, to even a minimally acceptable range of health services is a costly undertaking. Even were it possible to eliminate that part of cost stemming from unnecessary use, uneconomic operation and price escalation resulting from present provider reimbursement policies, if health services are made available to those who have hitherto been denied them for financial reasons, the total volume of service and thus of health expenditures will obviously rise, at least in the short run. In the longer run it is possible that earlier access to care and expansion of preventive services may reduce the need for service and thus costs (see below).

In recent years numerous health insurance bills have been introduced into Congress. All of them aim to remove or lower the financial barrier. But they differ greatly in how they propose to do so, and in the extent to which the barrier would be lowered.

A major difference among the proposals relates to the extent to which they contain provisions directed to assuring economy in the operation and in the use of resources and to the containment of price escalation. Another difference relates to the extent to which, and the manner in which, the various plans attempt to change the delivery system. Finally, there are significant differences in the arrangements for administration, as distinguished from the arrangements for the actual delivery of service. These administrative differences are revealed in the varying provisions made for the use or nonuse of private intermediaries or administrators, in the relative responsibilities assigned to the federal government and to the states, and in the role assigned to the consumer.[12]

## The Future

It is obvious that reform of the health services will be a major preoccupation of public policy in the years ahead. The problems to be solved are many and stubborn, and it would be hazardous to forecast what the system will look like by the year 2000. Yet some trends seem already evident.

### Lowering the Financial Barrier

First, there will be increased public action to remove or greatly lower the financial barrier to the receipt of medical care. Two policy issues will predominate: first, should publicly aided access to health services be assured on the basis of rights (through a free public service as in education or through social insurance), or should it be conditioned on individually demonstrated financial need? Second, how much of the financial barrier should be removed? The widespread dislike of a means- or income-tested system indicates that the trend will be toward a system conferring rights to health services. The size and diversity of the country and its limited experience with governmental involvement in the provision of financial support of personal health services suggests that for many years to come America will seek to secure these rights through the social insurance principle rather than through some form of national health service, although the latter would seem to be ultimately inevitable.

Adoption of the social insurance approach carries with it certain financial implications. If this technique is to remove or significantly lower the barrier for all or the vast majority of the population the contributions of the insured must be kept low. Already the Social Security taxes are scheduled to rise to 7.4% of wages (plus a similar percentage from the employer), and it is doubtful how much more regressive blood can be extracted from low-income stones, who are the very people for whom the financial burden is most acute. A sizable contribution from the general revenues will be essential.

If it is thought desirable that so far as possible the users of the service should carry some of its costs in order to strengthen cost-consciousness and foster self-restraint in its use or expansion, there will have to be a sharp distinction between payment of contributions as a partial source of financing and their payment as a determinant of eligibility. The application of insurance ideology, wherein payment of premiums serves as a device for excluding nonpayers from benefits, is inappropriate to a service which should be available to all with medical needs. It must become the responsibility of the general tax collector to ensure that all those required to pay taxes do so, but access to the service must not be dependent on having paid them. It is noteworthy that this policy is adopted in the Kennedy and Javits bills.

A second issue concerns the degree to which the financial barrier shall be removed: is it to be 100% of the average family's medical costs or some lesser percentage? Existing programs remove considerably less than 100% because only some kinds of medical care are included among the benefits and there are sizable deductions, copayments, and coinsurance. By 2000, and hopefully long before, it will surely have been realized, first, that such requirements are based on a false premise, namely that it is the patients rather than the professional providers (practitioners and institutions) who primarily determine how much and what kinds of care shall be received; and second, that such payments bear most heavily on the lower income receivers.[13] We can expect that deductibles will be restricted ultimately to a bare minimum and applied to cases where service demands are attributable to carelessness on the part of patients (e.g., loss of eyeglasses or dentures) or to optional procedures (e.g., cosmetic surgery).

Catastrophic health insurance is perhaps the approach which is calculated to do least to lower the financial barrier to needed care. In essence, it is an insurance program with high deductibles and copayment requirements so that reimbursement is available only after the patient has incurred sizable costs. Even then, reimbursement of excess costs is only partial, for such plans typically require coinsurance. Obviously the extent to which the financial burden on the patient is eased will depend upon the specific level of expenses the patient must carry himself before being eligible for some reimbursement, but the very terminology of such programs—"catastrophic" or "major medical"—implies that the level will be high. Thus, as in the 1971 Long bill, partial reimbursement would come into effect only after the patient himself had paid for the first 60 days of hospitalization and for $2,000 of physicians' or other types of health services, and the financial assistance to the average family would be small or, for low-income receivers, minuscule or zero. Most families with incomes under $6,000 or $7,000, let alone those in the $3,000-4,000 bracket, could not incur medical costs of even half those specified in the Long bill without acute hardship. In fact, catastrophic health insurance plans, where "catastrophic" is rigorously defined, are mainly of benefit to the rich. To benefit the nonrich it would be necessary to substitute for a uniform requirement of so many dollars of patient outlay, a measure that would define expenditures to be incurred in terms of some low percentage of a patient's income. Quite apart from the questionable policy of introducing what is in effect a form of income test, such a program would be administratively costly and cumbersome, especially if, as would seem logical, the qualifying percentage of income to be spent on medical care were to vary directly with the level of income.

Unfortunately, it seems probable that in the near future, some form of catastrophic health insurance will be enacted in the United States. Such a program would seem to have the political advantage of meeting the growing demand for national health insurance by adopting a system that will involve levying a minimum of additional federal taxation (for the less the burden removed from patients the less will the program "cost"). Such a plan, too, would seem to be a method of especially benefiting the nonaged middle classes who do not benefit from Medicare or Medicaid and who are now being pinched by escalating medical costs.

Yet it would seem inevitable that such a restricted form of national health insurance would be short-lived. On the one hand, its limited contribution to removal or lowering of the financial barrier would become increasingly apparent and give rise to pressure to lower the dollar cost-sharing requirement. But the lower the level of costs to be borne by the patient, the more such a program approaches the normal health insurance system with moderate cost-sharing requirements. On the other hand, a catastrophic insurance plan inevitably encourages cost escalation, and its operation would stimulate ever more rigorous efforts to control prices and utilization.

The extent to which any plan lowers the financial barrier to receipt of needed health services will also be affected by the range of services reimbursed or supplied. Determination of the scope of covered services will not be easy. Frequent references are made to "the basic health services" or to "acceptable minimal health services," but the components of these concepts remain to be defined. It would clearly be impractical, given limited manpower and institutional and equipment resources, to guarantee free or subsidized access to every type of care (e.g., heart transplants or kidney dialysis), and some would place long-term care in this category. But itemization of covered and uncovered services may distort treatment, lead to overuse of covered services, and run the risk of exclusion of important types of service. And of course all exclusions or durational limits will impose financial burdens on some types of patient. Since application of priorities will be essential, giving children a high priority for full service would make sense.

## Reform of the Delivery System

It is not difficult to forecast that a second trend will be a continuing search for a more effective delivery system. One that is acceptable implies an adequate and appropriately distributed supply of the various types of service providers both institutional and personal, and mechanisms to assure convenient access to primary care and effective linkages between the various forms or types of service needed by the individual patient. Of these, the problem of linkages is likely to be the most obstinate, although assuring a better distribution of medical personnel will not be easy.

Assurance of an adequate total supply of the various types of professional and paraprofessional personnel is likely to become increasingly a governmental responsibility. Private support for educational institutions, whether in the form of fees or philanthropic gifts, can no longer be relied on, except as a supplementary source of income. But increased governmental financial support will in time lead to increased governmental determination of the types of personnel whose education is to be publicly subsidized. This does not imply either monolithic control of all education for the health services or the elimination of all nongovernmental educational enterprise. But it does mean that there will be an acceptance of public responsibility for ensuring an adequate supply of the personnel needed to provide the range of services specified in the national plan, and a limitation of public subsidy to the production of such categories of personnel. Nor does this imply that the various professional and paraprofessional groups will exercise no influence over the determination of which categories shall receive public subsidy. On the contrary, the fierce competition among "disease specialists" (cancer, heart, etc.) for available public research funds in recent years suggests that the future may well see cleavages within the health professions and especially within the medical profession itself resulting from efforts by the different types of specialists and other providers to establish the essentiality of their particular expertise and the primacy of their claim to educational subsidies.

More difficult will be the problem of assuring an appropriate geographical distribution of the available total supply of personnel. Reliance on financial incentives or the possibility of repaying training loans or grants by defined periods of employment in underserviced areas appear to have only limited possibilities. To the extent that the relative isolation, in professional terms, of many rural areas deters physicians from practicing there, a better distribution of hospitals—especially teaching hospitals—with access to medical schools will ameliorate the situation. But more than this will be needed. Provision must be made for the rural practitioner's access to refresher courses and periodic contact with peers, including some who are better prepared or more up-to-date than he. An alternative approach can also be expected, namely experimentation with better communication and transport systems so as to bring the patient to the services he needs rather than, physically, bringing the services to him; this would also make available to the local practitioner consultation and associated diagnostic records. Shortage of personnel in the cities and especially in the ghetto areas cannot be thus explained and calls for different remedies. To the extent it is due to the lower economic capacity of the dwellers in these areas and thus a limitation on the earnings of physicians practicing therein, a national health insurance system would serve to make such areas financially more attractive. Indeed, Medicare and Medicaid have already made it profitable for physicians to relocate in certain poverty areas. Provision, through subsidy or direct leasing, of appropriate premises might also enhance the attractiveness of inner city areas as the locus of practice, as would assurance of access to, and staff privileges at, hospitals. In both rural and urban cases, perhaps in the end, America may have to adopt the British system of "negative control," whereby general practitioners may not enter practice under the public program in "overdoctored" areas, but this is likely to occur only as a last resort.[14]

Control over the proliferation and the location of various types of institutional facilities is already in effect in a limited number of areas and is likely to expand greatly in the years ahead, under the spur of cost containment. But this is largely a negative control directed to avoiding duplication or excessive concentration of facilities. There is need for equal attention to the problem of bringing into existence facilities of various types in areas where they are now lacking.

Reform of the delivery system involves more than assurance of an adequate and appropriately distributed supply of personnel and facilities. There is also a need to change the institutional structure through which services are delivered. Recognition of the importance of providing convenient access to primary care and assurance of subsequent linkages to other needed services has led to a revival of interest in prepaid group practice organizations. As envisaged today such an organization would undertake to provide, either itself or by contract with other providers such as hospitals, a specified range of services including prevention, diagnostic, treatment, hospitalization or other institutional care where indicated, and rehabilitation to an enrolled population who would pay an inclusive capitation fee. It would thus be in a position to provide the desired "one-door" access to all needed care.

Enthusiasm for this type of delivery unit is currently widespread, although it must be admitted that in some quarters its appeal seems to lie rather in the possibility that it may be a cheaper way of providing service rather than in its promise of better service. In any case, almost all health insurance proposals recently introduced included provisions aiming to encourage the formation of such organizations while the Nixon administration has made their promotion a major plank in its health reform program. It is however doubtful whether it is yet recognized how great an extension of public control over such models as the currently popular Health Maintenance Organizations (HMOs) will be inevitable if accountability is to be assured and if the interests of those who seek service and those who foot the bill are to be protected. Since the stimulus to their formation typically takes the form of generous financial aid and guarantees, there is a danger that profit-making groups may see a tempting opportunity for sizable profits at little risk. Not all the proposals limit participation to public or nonprofit corporations.[15] In view of the emphasis on economic operation and the offer of financial inducements to keep costs down, it will be necessary also to ensure that costs are not cut by poor service, discouragement of utilization of service or exclusion of bad risks. Consumers must be placed in a position to make choices, as between these provider systems and other delivery arrangements, by provision of adequate and widely distributed information regarding the services offered and the conditions attached thereto. Although the desirability of experimentation, pluralism and competition among providers is almost everywhere reiterated, it is questionable how many such competing delivery systems in any one community can be afforded, given the demands they will make on funds, organizing and management personnel and administrative supervision, or for that matter on discriminatory powers of consumers. Resolution of these problems would seem to make an extension of public standards and supervision inevitable.

Any rapid growth of such delivery systems is scarcely to be expected in view of the many technical problems involved in their organization, and current forecasts by Administration spokesmen would seem to be highly and overly optimistic. One obstacle will be the above-mentioned controls and constraints. For so long as the public program gives providers the option of reimbursement, even if functioning on a fee-for-service basis independently of such organizations, and thus not subject to these standards and supervisory controls, it seems likely that many will elect to remain imdependent, or, having joined, to withdraw from them, once the advantages of the subsidies and guarantees have been reaped.

It is indeed questionable whether, for the long run, an arrangement that permits both the prepaid group practice type of delivery system and independent fee-for-service "systems" will be viable. Its demise may well be hastened by the administrative complexity of dealing with thousands of independent providers in a world in which there will be on the one hand increasing pressure on government to check price escalation and on the other hand a growing demand from consumers for assurance of the quantity and quality of the services for which they have paid taxes.

In any case, experience has already shown that one of the obstacles to the growth of such organizations is the difficulty of attracting an enrollment adequate in size to provide a basis for economical operation. The existence of a comprehensive health insurance program would probably help to ameliorate this problem.

Yet even were all health services covered by the public program to be delivered through a network of HMO-type organizations, the task of reforming the delivery system would not be complete. Two major problems remain: assuring that the teaching hospitals and medical centers perform the functions which only they are equipped to perform but which are essential if high quality health services are to be rendered, and the development of appropriate organizations to supply certain services the need for which is common to all providers (HMOs or others) but which it would be uneconomic for each to provide for itself.

In the health service delivery system of the future the teaching hospitals and medical centers have an important role to play. Their role as undertakers of research is obvious and little difficulty is likely to be experienced in assuring that they continue to perform this function to the extent permitted by available public and philanthropic funds. The problem, in view of the emphasis on research and experimentation in medical technology in recent years, will rather be to ensure that they also accept other responsibilities.

The educational role of the hospitals and medical centers is long established and will obviously continue in future. Here the problem will be to ensure that appropriate provision is made for training for general practice and primary care, a field that has long been neglected in favor of an emphasis on specialization and intensive care. Community medicine is only slowly making its way into the curricula of the medical education system and still appears to be assigned little professional prestige. It is essential, too, that the medical centers and teaching hospitals of the future no longer confine their educational efforts to those who are formally enrolled in degree or graduate programs. As the repositories of scientific knowledge and the locus of technical experimentation, the hospitals need to be brought in touch with all the practitioners in their catchment areas. The need to upgrade the knowledge and skill of practitioners is increasingly apparent with the rapid advance of science and technology, and the hospitals have an important role to play, hopefully in cooperation with local medical societies, in preventing professional obsolescence. Similarly, the development of health resources within the community and the enhancement of standards in nursing homes and other types of extended care facilities are other areas where the hospitals could play a leadership role.

It is not easy to forecast what measures will be invented or utilized to ensure that the hospitals will in fact play the role that their unique and commanding position among the complex of service providers points to. One suggestion has been that hospitals participating in the public program should be franchised, and that the terms of the franchise would specify the types of service and responsibility which the hospital would agree to undertake.[16]

Reform of the delivery system also calls for arrangements to provide certain essential services needed by all providers whether operating independently or on a partnership or organized group practice basis, and which could either not be produced at all or operated only uneconomically by the providers themselves. These services, which I have called the health services infrastructure, include ambulance services, multiphasic screening facilities, laboratory testing over and above the most simple and routine procedures, maintenance of data banks and communication systems and the like. Some of these services are today provided on a competitive profit-making basis by the private sector. Yet it is difficult to see how wasteful use of the resources needed for their operation can be avoided and how access to these services can be assured to all providers in all parts of the country, or even within any one political jurisdiction, short of making their development and operation a public responsibility. Whether this should be a responsibility of the federal or of other levels of government would seem to depend on the nature of the service and the extent of its natural "market area." Thus ambulance services might well be operated by cities or counties or groups of these. On the other hand a data bank might ultimately cover the entire nation and thus become a federal responsibility.

### The Search for Appropriate Administrative Structures

The future administrative structure and the distribution of administrative functions among different agencies are not easy to forecast. Much will depend on the number and character of governmental programs in operation at any given time. The greater the number of public programs differing in their coverage and extent of services, in the principles underlying their eligibility conditions, in their methods of financing and in the agencies charged with their administration (public or private, and if public involving different levels of government), the more difficult will it be to ensure consistency of overall policy, appropriate coordination, avoidance of gaps in coverage and national accountability. It is to be hoped the number of different public programs will be reduced. In the meantime, the federal government could be expected to set a good example by introducing more order into the present complex and chaotic distribution of administrative responsibilities for the many health programs in which the federal government is involved.

Proposed health insurance systems such as those of Senators Kennedy and Javits would greatly reduce the number of different simultaneously operating public programs and bring into sharp focus

207

the need to determine an appropriate administrative structure for so large and comprehensive a program. Despite the currently popular use of the term "monolithic" in a pejorative sense, it seems inevitable that some administrative functions must be lodged in the federal government. They include the collection of revenues and their allocation among states, regions, groups of providers or specific components of the health system (such as provision of services, research, construction, education or training), specification of the minimum health benefits package, setting of standards of quality and for provider participation, coordinating any other health programs with which the federal government is involved and, above all, assuring fiscal and performance accountability. Only the federal government, too, has the data resources and the authority to prepare much-needed reports on the health status of the nation as a whole and on major unmet needs. There would seem to be much merit in the proposal for lodging this last function in a National Health Council, similar in status and administrative location to the Council of Economic Advisers, which would also be charged with the duty of making recommendations for policy changes.

But it does not follow that all of the day-to-day administering and on-the-spot monitoring of the providers of service would have to be done by federal officials. There is much to be said for involving the states.

The desirability of as much devolution as possible in a national program concerned with the provision of services rather than cash payments, the fact that many health or health-related functions are already located in the states, and the probability that, at least initially, the national health package will be limited, thus enhancing the desirability of allowing leeway for additional benefits provided by states willing and able to do so—all these suggest the wisdom of retaining the states in the administrative structure. For regional or other nonpolitical administrative units have neither a political base nor fund-raising capacity. The states could be involved through contracts with the federal government to perform specified functions (including establishment of intrastate or interstate regions) in conformity with federal criteria and standards. But in the event of inability or unwillingness of a state to sign such a contract, or having done so to live up to it, it would be necessary to ensure that administrative responsibilities would revert to the federal government.

For the longer run it seems likely that the administrative role of private insurance companies will be minimal or zero. As governments gain administrative experience the necessity for their use will be less apparent, the increased measure of public control over their activities which will be necessary if accountability, quality of service, cost containment and consumer satisfaction are to be assured may well make participation less attractive to the companies themselves. It also seems inevitable that with the passage of time, the inappropriateness of the underlying concepts of the private profit-making insurance approach to assurance of adequate universally available health services will become increasingly apparent.

Finally, it is not difficult to forecast that the administrative arrangements of the future will include a vastly broadened role for the consumer—another reason for restricting the role of private insurance companies for in a complex service such as health adequate consumer influence is not assured merely by competition among providers. The years ahead will undoubtedly see a variety of experiments with a view to identifying those aspects of a health service program with which the consumer should appropriately be involved either in an advisory capacity or in decision-making, to determining the points in the administrative or delivery system at which consumer participation would be most effective and to the selection and staff-servicing of appropriate consumer representatives.

### The Costs of the Health Services

At least one forecast can be made with considerable confidence: the costs of the health services will continue to rise. When the word "costs" is used in connection with proposals for new methods of financing and organizing health services, it usually refers to the additional taxation any given plan would involve, and there is a tendency to evaluate its desirability by reference to its "costs" in this sense. The impression is thus given that the program in question imposes a new burden on income-receivers. In fact, except for possible increases in total national health expenditures due to the provision of services to people previously denied them for financial reasons, or to expanded or irresponsible use of services which have become free or subsidized (see below), all proposals merely change the allocation of costs already being carried, i.e., they are another way of paying for an existing bill.[17] For while income receivers as a group will pay more as federal taxpayers (through earmarked social insurance contributions or through income or other taxes), they will pay less for their health services as patients, as purchasers of private health insurance or as state and local taxpayers supporting Medicaid.

This change in allocation of health costs may take two forms: one highly visible, one less so. The visible effect is obtained when new or

209

additional taxes are imposed specifically to finance the proposed program, as would be the case with the Long, the Kennedy and the Javits bills as well as the Nixon federally subsidized Family Health Insurance plan. The transfer is less visible and the cost apt to be underestimated when, as in the proposals of the AMA or the HIAA or the Byrnes version of the Nixon plan, employers or individuals are allowed to credit the health insurance premiums they pay against their federal tax obligations. For the effect on the federal tax-payer is the same, because the revenue lost because of the tax credit or deduction must be recouped by increased taxes on federal tax-payers as a group. Whether the cost of any proposal is high or low depends on how much of the burden of health care expenditures now carried by users of the services is reallocated. A limited program applicable to only some types of health service or covering relatively few people or reimbursing only a small fraction of patient expenditures will have a low "cost": conversely, one that is comprehensive in terms of population and service coverage will have a high "cost." Thus the Long bill, which is essentially a catastrophic insurance plan with deductibles so high that relatively few patients will qualify for even partial reimbursement, obviously increases the financial burden on the taxpayer only slightly (by $3.1 billions according to the estimates of the government actuary[18]). The Nixon family plan which would subsidize the costs of a limited health insurance system restricted to the poor nonemployed would also involve a low ($3.06) burden on the federal taxpayer.

On the other hand, the Kennedy bill, which would increase the need for federal taxation by the largest amount (estimated at $59.4 billions), would do so because it would give greater financial relief to a vastly larger number of individual patients, purchasers of private health insurance and state and local taxpayers. Similarly, the Javits bill, which is only somewhat less comprehensive than the Kennedy bill, would have a high "cost" ($41.6 billions).

But there is another and more significant meaning of the word "costs," namely, as measuring the total national expenditure on the health services. Costs in this sense can be expected to rise in the years ahead as they have risen in the past. Even with no change in methods of financing and delivery sheer population growth will mean, if levels of quality and availability of service are to remain as at present, that a greater volume of resources must be devoted to the health services. This would not necessarily mean that such expenditures would account for a larger percentage of the Gross National Product (the nation's total output), for this is also likely to increase in the future. But it is probable that on a per capita basis too (i.e., making allowance for population growth), expenditures will rise because of the availability of new and more costly medical technologies, procedures, and techniques and other new inputs in the health services.[19] Furthermore, if past experience is a guide, expenditures will continue to rise because of the increase in prices charged by providers.[20] Nor does it seem likely that there will be any abatement of the long secular increase in the demand for services on the part of consumers who have high expectations of what modern medicine can accomplish and thus value the services more highly.

It is factors such as these that account for the impressive increase in total health expenditures over the last forty years. As is shown in Table 1, the increase has occurred not only in national totals but also in terms of expenditures per capita and as a percentage of Gross National Product. Even more startling, perhaps, is the estimate of the Actuary of the Social Security Administration that assuming no further legislation changing the financing or administration of the health services, national expenditures by 1974 may well reach $105 billions[21].

Changes in methods of financing and organization will of course have an impact on total expenditures, although their extent is difficult to estimate. On the one hand expenditures will rise to the extent that the new programs, by lowering the financial barrier, permit people who were previously unable to use the services, henceforth to enjoy them. Furthermore, some additional usage may well result from the fact that when a good or service is free or heavily subsidized, peeople will use more of it or use it less responsibly. In addition, if the new arrangements necessitate larger organizing or administrative staffs than the previous system, costs will again rise. But on the other hand, costs may decline if, by making more visible the extent of rising expenditures, the new arrangements stimulate effective measures to control or at least put a brake on price escalation, and to encourage greater efficiency of operation and more economical use of manpower, technical equipment and capital resources. It is possible, too, that administrative costs may be lower than before (consider, for example, the administrative economies of collecting health insurance premiums through existing federal tax machinery as compared with the employment of commissioned agents by competitive private insurance companies). Finally, if the new arrangements serve to encourage greater development of preventive health services, either deliberately due to a concern about cost cutting or because patients are more likely to seek early diagnosis and treatment when undeterred by financial considerations, they will tend to lower expenditures—at least in the longer run.

**Table 1: National Health Expenditures**
**(Selected fiscal years 1929-1971)**

| Fiscal Year | Total (in $ millions) | Per Capita | Percent of GNP |
|---|---|---|---|
| 1928-29 | 3,589 | 29.16 | 3.6 |
| 1939-40 | 3,863 | 28.83 | 4.1 |
| 1949-50[a] | 12,028 | 78.35 | 4.6 |
| 1959-60 | 25,857 | 141.61 | 5.2 |
| 1964-65[b] | 38,892 | 197.81 | 5.9 |
| 1966-67 | 49,860 | 237.93 | 6.2 |
| 1969-70 | 67,770 | 326.78 | 7.1 |
| 1970-71 | 75,012 | 358.05 | 7.4 |

[a] immediately prior to the Social Security Amendments of 1950 authorizing federal sharing in vendor payments.

[b] immediately prior to enactment of Medicare and Medicaid.

Source: Cooper, BS, Worthington NL: *National Health Expenditures, Fiscal Year 1971*, Research and Statistics Note No. 13-1971, Social Security Administration, Department of HEW, Washington, D.C., November 19, 1971.

It seems likely that the final balance of these forces will result in a national expenditure that will be larger than would have occurred in the absence of new legislation, if only because the one certain outcome of all proposed changes will be some increase in the numbers of people receiving care and/or in the range of services received by many people. However, the increase in total expenditures is unlikely to be enormous in relation to that which is likely to occur in any case. The federal actuary has estimated that total national expenditures by 1974 under the various health insurance bills before the Congress in 1971 would range from $106.5 billions to $116.8 billions.[22]

In any case, the totals are large and raise in the minds of many people a question: Can they be afforded? When considering how much a society can afford to spend on any given group of goods and services, it is important to bear in mind that the dollar figures are only a convenient way of measuring the volume of basic economic resources (labor, capital equipment, organizing ability and the like) embodied in their production. At any given time the total volume of productive resources available to the nation is limited.[23] If used to produce health services these resources cannot be used to produce something else. Thus the "cost" of the health services is the alternative products that could have been produced by the resources devoted to the health services.

Within the limits of the total productive resources available to the nation therefore, it is not a matter of economics but of choices and values as to how much shall be devoted to the health services and how much to the production of houses or TV sets or automobiles or household gadgets or day care centers or schools and the like. As Table 1 shows, the nation has come to attach an increasingly high relative value to health services as evidenced by the ever-increasing percentage of Gross National Product devoted to this end. Whether this trend will continue will depend on psychological and political factors. It will depend, on the one hand, on the intensity of dissatisfaction on the part of the electorate with present arrangements for the financing and organization of the health services and, on the other, on the willingness of federal taxpayers to allow their Congress to enact additional taxes in return for a reduction of their personal expenditures on the health services, as patients, purchasers of private health insurance and as state and local taxpayers supporting such programs as Medicaid. The outcome will be the more uncertain in that this kind of *quid pro quo* will not be experienced equally by all federal taxpayers. For the poor cannot contribute their proportionate share of the costs and the gap must be filled by more than proportionate contributions (i.e., taxes) from higher income receivers. Some measure of income redistribution is thus inevitably involved, and what happens in the end will depend on values and attitudes toward the desirability of a more equalitarian society.

However, if as this writer believes, the trend will be toward the adoption of ever more comprehensive measures to remove the financial barrier and to change the delivery system, with resulting increases in expenditures, it does not follow that nothing can be done to contain costs. A rational society would surely aim to ensure that any given volume or level of health services utilizes as few resources as possible, thereby maximizing those available for other uses. In the years ahead, what can realistically be expected are more concentrated and sophisticated efforts to ensure more economical use and provision of health services. One line of attack will be a more rigorous effort to limit price escalation and much experimentation with techniques and incentives can be expected. It seems likely, however, that even by the year 2000 the problem of the remuneration of providers will be unsolved. Financial arrangements that satisfy both providers and those who foot the bill are not easily found, as the experience of countries with long-established health insurance or national health services demonstrates. It seems inevitable that there will be a much greater use of the capitation system applicable to groups of professional providers and it may well be that ultimately the publicly financed or subsidized system will deny participation to professionals who engage in solo practice on a fee-for-service basis. Although such a development would be strongly opposed by some members of organized medicine, both the administrative complexities of dealing with hundreds and thousands of individual providers and the impossibility of assuring comprehensive and continuous care when service is provided on an item-by-item, fee-for-service basis will be strong forces making for change.

Undoubtedly too, there will be more extensive and rigorous controls, including the strengthening of the capacity and authority of planning bodies at all levels, over the location, expansion and administrative operation of hospitals and other institutional facilities.[24] There will be increasing efforts to avoid duplication or underutilization of expensive facilities and equipment where supply is excessive in relation to the needs of any given area. Undoubtedly, too, there will be an expansion of the availability and use of the less expensive forms of institutional care, and where feasible, the substitution of institutional care by other services which make possible care in the home.

These efforts to evaluate and constrain the prices charged by, and to improve the efficiency of operation of, the various types of providers, personal and institutional, will necessitate the creation of a highly skilled corps of technical experts. These are in very short supply and as yet neither schools of administrative medicine nor departments of economics have adequately responded to the challenge to produce more of them. It is important to note that the need for this kind of expertise is not created by the passage of health insurance legislation. Concern about costs, prices, efficiency and the reasonableness of charges is experienced also by private insurance companies, by hospitals and by medical societies all of whom in future will need the assistance of sophisticated technical personnel.

The aim of cost containment will also foster intensified efforts to increase the supply and encourage the use of paraprofessional and auxiliary personnel.

Greater emphasis on health education is to be anticipated. This is not merely a matter of transmitting to an increasingly better educated population more knowledge of the functioning of the body and of symptoms and simple forms of self-medication and knowledge of when to consult professionals. More importantly, and more difficult to achieve, it involves educating the consumer in the principles of healthy living in regard to such matters as nutrition, smoking, exercise and the like.

It will surely be realized, too, in the years ahead, that expenditures on the health services can be contained by reducing the need for them through action in areas other than those classified as "health." Greater knowledge of the health effects of environmental pollution, low incomes, poor housing, conditions of employment or unwanted pregnancies will surely lead to a recognition that additional dollars invested in the elimination of these evils will often be more productive than investment of additional dollars in the traditional health services.

## Notes

1. *Medical Care for the American People.* The Final Report of the Committee on the Costs of Medical Care (adopted October 31, 1932): 32-34. The report was republished by the US Department of Health, Education and Welfare, Public Health Service (1970). Washington, DC, Government Printing Office.

2. See Note 1, Chapter 9.

3. The proportion of personal health expenditures met through private insurance rose from 8.3% in fiscal 1950 to 23.8% in fiscal 1970. For the current extent of private health insurance, see Mueller MS: Private health insurance in 1969: A review." *Social Security Bulletin* 34 (February, 1971); 3-18.

4. For an account of the obstacles to the growth of prepaid group practice and extensive references see Greenberg IG, Rodburg, ML: The role of prepaid group practice in relieving the medical care crisis." *Harvard Law Review,* 84 (February, 1971); 887-1001, especially Part IV. A briefer account is given in Bush AS: *Group Practice.* New York State Health Planning Commission, Office of Planning Sources, New York, September 1971.

5. Apart from expansions of the traditional public health services and public support of care for the needy, it had envisaged only limited subsidies from public funds to the voluntary health insurance premiums of low income families, the use of tax funds for local hospital services and for institutional care of chronic diseases. The majority held that the larger units of government should be involved only when it was evident that smaller units were financially incompetent.

6. For the extent of governmental responsibilities by 1970 see Chapter 2.

7. Rice D., and Cooper B.: National health expenditures (1929-70). *Social Security Bulletin,* XXXIV, 1 (January 1971), 5, 15; Cooper BS, Worthington N: National Health Expenditures, (1929-71). *Social Security Bulletin, XXXV,* 1, 5, 13.

8. See Note 2 above.

9. Even the addition in 1967 of a provision limiting "prevailing charges" to the level necessary to embrace the 75th percentile of customary charges in the physicians locality has not succeeded in stemming the upward trend of charges.

10. As late as 1972, federal auditors were reporting serious business inefficiencies and overpayments to doctors on the part of insurance companies and Blue Shield in a number of states. *New York Times,* March 8, 1972.

11. P.L. 92-603 mandated the payment of premiums by the medically needy and permitted the imposition of deductibles and copayments on both them and, for optional services, on cash assistance recipients. Also, the requirement that by 1977 a state must have a comprehensive program covering all needy and medically indigent persons was eliminated as was the "maintenance of effort" requirement.

12. For details see Chapters 8 and 9.

13. A survey conducted by Blue Cross and Blue Shield among all United States plans on the effectiveness of deductibles, coinsurance and copayments in 1971 revealed a remarkable consensus to the effect that the nature of their impact on unnecessary utilization was "hazy," that they would act as a barrier to needed care, and that if lowered sufficiently not to create hardship they became "nothing more than administrative nuisances." They were stigmatized as a hoped-for "easy answer" to cost control to avoid contending with the much more difficult problem of dealing with the doctor and his style of medical practice. Blue Cross and Blue Shield, *Report on Deductibles, Coinsurance and Copayments.* Chicago, September 1971 Mimeographed.

14. In Great Britain, control over the geographic distribution of specialists is

215

assured because of their employment by the government-owned hospitals, so that it is the government that ultimately controls hospital staffing through approval of budgets.

15. The recipients of $65.5 million planning grants in fiscal 1971 included physician groups, medical schools, neighborhood health centers, community hospitals, medical societies, state and local health departments and private corporations. *Group Health and Welfare News,* August, 1971, 8.

16. Somers AR: *Health Care in Transition: Directions for the Future.* Chicago, Chicago Hospital and Educational Trust, 1971.

17. Thus some current proposals would transfer expenditure from individual purchasers of care to employers by requiring employers to provide specified health benefits as a fringe benefit, or to the general taxpayer through subsidies to a compulsory or voluntary health insurance plan, or to the group of insured people as a whole through the payment of compulsory health insurance contributions (or taxes).

18. These and the following estimates are from *Analysis of Health Insurance Proposals Introduced in the 92nd Congress,* printed for the use of the Committee on Ways and Means, Committee Print, 92nd Cong, 1st Sess, August 1971. Washington, DC, Government Printing Office.

19. It has been estimated that of the increase in hospital costs per patient day from $16.77 in 1951 to $81.01 in 1970, 50.6% was attributable to new inputs such as new technology, techniques, new and expensive drugs and new and costly procedures such as open heart surgery and to additional services such as new parking spaces, remodelled waiting rooms, improved quality of food served, etc. Waldman S: *The Effect of Changing Technology on Hospital Costs.* Research and Statistics Notes, No. 4, Social Security Administration, HEW, February 28, 1972.

20. It has been estimated that between 1966 and 1970, rising prices accounted for the following proportions of increasing expenditures: on hospital care, 76.3%; on physicians' services, 69.1%; and on dental services, 58.9%. Rice DP, and Cooper BS: *op cit,* 10-13.

21. *Analysis of Health Insurance Proposals Introduced in the 92nd Congress, loc cit,* 81.

22. *Ibid,* 76.

23. To the extent that there are unutilized resources—due to unemployment, for example—additional health services could be provided without reducing the production of other goods and services. Even so, there is still the possibility that these unused resources might have been used to produce additional consumer goods other than health services.

24. The problems of controlling hospital costs are explored in Somers AR: *Hospital Regulation: The Dilemma of Public Policy,* New Jersey, Industrial Relations Section, Princeton University, 1969; Somers HM, AR: *Medicare and the Hospitals: Issues and Prospects.* Washington, DC, the Brookings Institution, 1967.

# Selected Bibliography

The literature dealing with the problems of the health services has been so voluminous in recent years that a comprehensive bibliography would almost form a separate book. In what follows I have selected books and reports bearing directly on the subject matter of this book which I have found especially useful or which contain extensive bibliographies. Students of the health services would do well to consult the long series of Congressional Hearings on health legislation and related problems. These Hearings contain not only full explanations of proposed legislation but also the viewpoints of the Administration, of organized interest groups, both professional and lay, and of individual experts. In addition, they include much statistical and other data not otherwise readily available, and frequently also reprints of important articles and reports. Among the more informative are the following:

US, Congress, House, Subcommittee of Committee on Government Operations, *Administration of Federal Health Benefit Programs, Hearings,* 91st Cong., 2nd sess. Washington, DC, US Government Printing Office, 1970.

US, Congress, Senate, Committee on Appropriations, *Departments of Labor and Health, Education, and Welfare, Appropriations Fiscal Year 1971,* HR 18515, 91st Cong., 2nd sess., Part 4 . Washington, DC, US Government Printing Office, 1970.

US, Congress, Senate, Committee on Finance, *Social Security,* Hearings on HR 6675, 89th Cong., 1st sess. Washington, DC, US Government Printing Office, 1965.

US, Congress, Senate, Committee on Finance, *Social Security Amendments of 1971, Hearings,* 92nd Cong., 1st and 2nd sess. Washington, DC, US Government Printing Office, 1972.

US, Congress, Senate, *Committee on Government Operations, Health Care in America,* Subcommittee on Executive Reorganization, 90th Cong., 2nd sess. Washington, DC, US Government Printing Office, 1968.

US, Congress, Senate, Committee on Government Operations, *Federal Role in*

*Health,* Report No. 91-809, 91st Cong., 2nd sess. Washington, DC, US Government Printing Office, 1970.

US, Congress, Senate, Committee on the Judiciary, · Subcommittee on Anti-trust and Monopoly, *High Cost of Hospitalization,* 91st Cong., 2nd sess. Washington, DC, US Government Printing Office, 1971.

US, Congress, Senate, Committee on Labor and Public Welfare, *National Health Insurance,* Hearings on S 4323 and S 3830, 91st Cong., 2nd sess. Washington, DC, US Government Printing Office, 1970.

US, Congress, Senate, Committee on Labor and Public Welfare, Subcommittee on Health, *Health Care Crisis in America, Hearings,* 92nd Cong., 1st sess. Washington, DC, US Government Printing Office, 1971.

US, Congress, Senate, Committee on Labor and Public Welfare, Subcommittee on Health, *Physicians Training Facilities and Health Maintenance Organizations,* Hearings on S 935, S 703, S 837, S 1182, S 1301, 92nd Cong., 1st sess. Washington, DC, US Government Printing Office, 1971.

US, Congress, Senate, Committee on Labor and Public Welfare, Subcommittee on Health, *Physicians Training Facilities and Health Maintenance Organizations,* Hearings on S 935, S 703, S 387, S 1182, S 1301, S 2827, S 3327, 92nd Cong., 1st and 2nd sess. Washington, DC, US Government Printing Office, 1971, 1972.

The following references do not include articles (many of which are referred to in footnotes in the preceding chapters) except articles that are comprehensive reports on special topics.

## Historical and General

*The American Medical Association; Power, Purpose and Politics in Organized Medicine. Yale Law Journal,* Vol 63, 1954.

Anderson OW: *The Uneasy Equilibrium; Private and Public Financing of Health Services in the United States, 1875–1965.* New Haven, College and University Press, 1968.

Corning PA: *The Evolution of Medicare.* US Department of Health, Education and Welfare, Social Security Administration, Research Report No 29. Washington, DC, US Government Printing Office, 1969.

Freeman RB: *Community Health Nursing Practice.* Philadelphia, W. B. Saunders, 1970.

Health Services Research, New York. *Milbank Memorial Fund Quarterly,* Vol 44, No 3, July 1966, and No. 4, October 1966.

*Hill-Burton Program: Progress Report 1947–1965.* Public Health Service, US Department of Health, Education, and Welfare. Washington, DC, Health Service, 1965.

Klarman HE: *The Economics of Health.* New York, Columbia University Press, 1965.

*Medical Care in Transition: Reprints from the American Journal of Public Health.* Vol I, 1949–1957, Vol II, 1958–1962. US Department of Health, Education and Welfare, Public Health Service. Washington, DC, US Government Printing Office, 1964.

Rosen G: *A History of Public Health.* New York, Schumann, 1958.

Rosenberg K, Schiff G: *The Politics of Health Care: A Bibliography.* Boston, New England Free Press, 1972.

Scott WR, Volkart, EH, editors: *Medical Care: Readings in the Sociology of Medical Institutions.* New York, John Wiley & Sons, 1966.

Shyrock RH: *The History of Nursing: An Interpretation of the Social and Medical Factors Involved.* Philadelphia, W.B. Saunders, Co 1959.

Somers HM, Somers AR: *Doctors, Patients and Health Insurance: The Organization and Financing of Medical Care.* Washington, DC, The Brookings Institution, 1961.

Stevens R: *American Medicine and the Public Interest.* New Haven, Yale University Press, 1971.

US, Congress, Senate, Subcommittee of the Committee on Education and Labor, *To Establish a National Health Program,* Hearings on S 1620, 76th Cong., 1st sess. Washington, DC, US Government Printing Office, 1939.

US, Congress Senate, Committee on Education and Labor, *Medical Care Insurance: A Social Insurance Plan for Personal Health Services.* Committee Print No. 5, 79th Cong., 2nd sess. Washington, DC, US Government Printing Office, 1946.

US, Department of Health, Education, and Welfare, *Proceedings of the White House Conference on Health, November 1965.* Washington, DC, US Government Printing Office, 1965.

US, Department of Health, Education, and Welfare, Public Health Service, *Medical Care for the American People.* The Final Report of the Committee on the Costs of Medical Care, 1932. Washington, DC, US Government Printing Office, 1970.

US, President's Commission on the Health Needs of the Nation, *Building America's Health: A Report to the President.* 5 vol. Washington, DC, US Government Printing Office, 1952, 1953.

## Today's Health Services

American Medical Association, Center for Health Services, Research and Development: *Reference Data on Socio-economic Issues of Health, 1971.* Chicago, American Medical Association, 1971.

Anderson OW: *Health Services in a Land of Plenty.* Chicago, University of Chicago Press, 1968.

Annals of the American Academy of Political and Social Science. *The Nation's Health,* Vol 399, January 1972, entire issue.

Closing the Gaps in the Availability and Accessibility of Health Services. The 1965 Health Conference of the New York Academy of Medicine, New York. *Bulletin of the New York Acadmey of Medicine,* Vol 41, No 12, December 1965.

*Community Health Services for New York City.* Report and Staff Studies of the Commission on the Delivery of Personal Health Services. New York, Praeger, 1969.

Conference on Health Services for Children and Youth. Supplement. *American Journal of Public Health,* Vol 60, No 4, April 1970.

Fuchs VC, editor: *Essays in the Economics of Health and Medical Care.* New York, The National Bureau of Economic Research, 1972.

Ginsberg E, Ostow M: *Men, Money and Medicine.* New York, Columbia University Press, 1969.

*Health is A Community Affair.* Report of the National Commission on Community Health Services. Cambridge, Harvard University Press, 1967.

Health Insurance Institute: *Source Book of Health Insurance Data.* New York, Health Insurance Institute, annually.

Joint Commission on Mental Illness and Health: *Action for Mental Health, Final Report.* New York, Basic Books, 1961.

Jones B, editor: *The Health of Americans.* New York, The American Assembly, 1970.

Kennedy EM: *In Critical Condition–The Crisis in America's Health Care.* New York, Simon and Schuster, 1972.

Kosa J, Antonovsky A, Antonovsky Z, et al, editors: *Poverty and Health.* Cambridge, Harvard University Press, 1969.

Kramer MS, Kramer C: Fragmented Financing of Health Care. *Medical Care Review,* Vol 29, No 8. (August 1972) pp 878–943.

La Rocco A, editor: *Poverty and Health in the United States, A Bibliography with Abstracts.* New York, Medical and Health Research Association of New York City, 1967.

*Maternal and Child Health Program, A Program Analysis.* Washington, DC, US Department of Health, Education, and Welfare, 1966.

*Medical Care Prices: A Report to the President.* US Department of Health, Education, and Welfare, February 1967. Washington, DC, US Government Printing Office, 1967.

Medical Industrial Complex. *Health-Pac Bulletin.* New York, Health Policy Advisory Center, November 1969.

Neighborhood Health Centers. *Medical Care,* Vol 8, No 2, March-April, 1970, entire issue.

Perrott GS: *The Federal Employees Health Benefits Program: Enrollment and Utilization of Health Service 1961-1968.* US Department of Health, Education and Welfare, Health Services and Mental Health Administration, 1971.

Piore N, Lewis D, Seelinger J: *A Statistical Profile of Hospital Outpatients Services in the United States.* New York, Association for the Aid of Crippled Children, 1971.

Reed LS, Carr W: *The Benefit Structure of Private Health Insurance, 1968.* Social Security Administration, US Department of Health, Education and Welfare, Research Report No 32. Washington, DC, US Government Printing Office, 1970.

*Report of the National Advisory Commission on Health Manpower.* Two volumes. Washington, DC, US Government Printing Office, 1967.

*Secretary's Advisory Committee on Hospital Effectiveness–Report.* US Department of Health, Education, and Welfare. Washington, DC, US Government Printing Office, 1968.

*Social Policy for Health Care.* Papers presented to the Subcommittee on Social Policy for Health Care, of the Committee on Special Studies. New York, The New York Academy of Medicine, 1969.

Somers HM, Somers AR: *Private Health Insurance, Parts I and II.* Institute of Industrial Relations, Reprints No 113 and No 118. Berkeley, University of California, 1958.

*The Family Doctor. Milbank Memorial Fund Quarterly,* Vol I, No 2, entire issue. *New York: April 1972, Part 2.*

US, Congress, House, Committee on Ways and Means, *Basic Facts on the Health Industry,* a Staff Report. Committee Print, 92nd Cong., 1st sess., 1971. Washington, DC, US Government Printing Office, 1971.

US, Department of Health, Education, and Welfare. *Human Investment Programs: Delivery of Health Services to the Poor.* Washington, DC, US Government Printing Office, 1967.

US, Department of Health, Education, and Welfare, Social Security Administration, *Medical Care Costs and Prices: Background Book.* Washington, DC, January 1972.

US, National Advisory Commission on Health Facilities, *Report.* Washington, DC, US Government Printing Office, 1968.

See also Congressional Hearings cited above.

## Medicare and Medicaid

Somers AR: *Hospital Regulation: The Dilemma of Public Policy.* Princeton, Industrial Relations Section, 1969.

Somers HM, Somers AR: *Medicare and the Hospitals.* Washington, DC, Brookings Institution, 1967.

US, Congress, Senate, Committee on Finance, *Medicare and Medicaid:* A Staff Report, 91st Cong., 1st sess. Washington, DC, US Government Printing Office, 1970.

Congress, Senate, Committee on Finance, *Medicare and Medicaid: Hearings,* 91st Cong., 1st sess. Washington, DC, US Government Printing Office, 1969.

US, Congress, Senate, Committee on Finance, *Medicare and Medicaid: Hearings,* 91st Cong., 2nd sess. Washington, DC, US Government Printing Office, 1970.

US, Department of Health, Education, and Welfare, *Report of the Task Force on Medicaid and Medicare.* Washington, DC, US Government Printing Office, 1970.

US, Department of Health, Education, and Welfare, Social Security Administration. *Financing Mental Health Care under Medicare and Medicaid.* Research Report No. 37. Washington, DC, US Government Printing Office, 1971.

# Prepaid Group Practice

Feldstein P: *Prepaid Group Practice: An Analysis and Review.* Ann Arbor, Michigan University Bureau of Hospital Administration, 1971.

Group Practice: Problems and Perspectives. The 1968 Health Conference of the New York Academy of Medicine, New York: *Bulletin of the New York Academy of Medicine,* Vol 44, No 11, November 1968.

*Promoting the Group Practice of Medicine.* Report of the National Conference on Group Practice, US Department of Health, Education, and Welfare, Washington, DC, October, 1967.

MacColl WA: *Group Practice and Prepayment of Medical Care.* Washington, DC, Public Affairs Press, 1966.

Somers AR, editor: *The Kaiser-Permanente Medical Care Program, A Symposium.* New York, The Commonwealth Fund, 1971.

# Manpower

*Education for the Allied Health Professions and Services.* US Department of Health, Education, and Welfare, Public Health Service Publication No 1600, Washington, DC, 1967.

Fein R: *The Doctor Shortage: An Economic Diagnosis.* Washington, DC, The Brookings Institution, 1967.

*Health Manpower, Employment Service Review,* Vol 3, No 11, November 1966, entire issue. US Department of Labor, Bureau of Employment Security. Washington, DC, US Government Printing Office, 1966.

*Health Manpower: Factors of Crisis.* A reprint of articles from *Medical Tribune,* North Miami General Hospital, North Miami. 1968.

*Higher Education and the Nation's Health.* Report and Recommendations by the Carnegie Commission on Higher Education. New York, McGraw-Hill, 1970.

*Physicians for a Growing America.* Report of the Surgeon General's Consultant Group on Medical Education, US Department of Health, Education, and Welfare, Public Health Service. Washington, DC, US Government Printing Office, 1959.

*Reports of the National Advisory Commission on Health Manpower.* Two Volumes. Washington, DC, US Government Printing Office, 1967.

Sadler AM Jr, Sadler BL, Bliss AA: *The Physician's Assistant: Today and Tomorrow.* New Haven, Yale University Press, 1972.

*Training Health Service Workers: The Critical Challenge.* Conference Proceedings, US Department of Labor and US Department of Health, Education, and Welfare. Washington, DC, US Government Printing Office, 1966.

*The Fuller Utilization of the Woman Physician.* Report of a Conference on Meeting Medical Manpower Needs. Washington, DC, US Department of Labor, Women's Bureau, 1966.

*The Graduate Education of Physicians.* Report of the Citizens' Commission on Graduate Medical Education, The Council on Medical Education, American Medical Association, Chicago, n.d.

222

# Proposals for Reform

American Medical Association, Division of Medical Practice, *Health Maintenance Organizations as Seen by the American Medcial Association: An Analysis.* Chicago: American Medical Association, 1971.

*Ameriplan: A Proposal for the Delivery and Financing of Health Services in the US* Report of a special committee on the Provision of Health Services, American Hospital Association, Chicago, 1970.

*A Report to the President on Medical Care Prices, 1967.* US Department of Health, Education, and Welfare. Washington, D.C.

Brewster AW: *Health Insurance and Related Proposals for Financing Personal Health Services: A Digest of Major Legislation and Proposals for Federal Action 1935–1957.* US Department of Health, Education, and Welfare, Social Security Administration, Washington, DC, 1958.

*Comprehensive Health Planning: A Selected Annotated Bibliography.* Publication No 1953. Washington, DC, US Public Health Service, 1967.

"Creative Federalism"; "Partnership in Health"; Slogans or Solutions? The 1969 Health Conference of the New York Academy of Medicine. *Bulletin of the New York Academy of Medicine,* 1969.

Davis MM: *America Organizes Medicine.* New York, Harper & Bros., 1941.

*Ibid. Medical Care for Tomorrow.* New York, Harper & Bros., 1955.

Eilers RD, Moyerman SS, editors: *National Health Insurance.* Proceedings of the Conference on National Health Insurance, Homewood, Illinois, Richard D. Irwin, 1971.

Falk IS: *National Policies and Programs for the Financing of Medical Care.* The Michael M. Davis Lecture Series 9. Chicago, Center for Health Administration Studies, University of Chicago, 1971.

*Financing Health Maintenance Care and Delivery.* New York, New York National Association of Manufacturers, n.d.

Follman JF: *Medical care and Health Insurance.* Homewood, Illinois, Richard D. Irwin, 1963.

National Commission on Community Health Services: *Health Administration and Organization in the Decade Ahead.* Washington, DC, Public Affairs Press, 1967.

New Directions in Public Policy for Health Care. The 1966 Health Conference of the New York Academy of Medicine, New York. *Bulletin of the New York Academy of Medicine,* Vol 42, No 12, December 1966.

*Reimbursement Incentives for Hospital and Medical Care: Objectives and Alternatives.* Social Security Administration, Department of Health, Education, and Welfare, Research Report No 26, Washington, DC, US Government Printing Office, 1968.

New York State: *Report from the Governor's Steering Committee on Social Problems on Health and Hospital Services and Costs.* New York, 1971.

.*Rx for Action.* Report of the Health Task Force of the Urban Coalition. Washington, DC, The Urban Coalition, n.d.

Somers AR: *Health Care in Transition: Directions for the Future.* Chicago, Hospital Research and Educational Trust, 1971.

Somers AR: *Hospital Regulation: The Dilemma of Public Policy,* Princeton, Princeton University, 1969.

US, Congress, House, Committee on Interstate and Foreign Commerce, Subcommittee on Public Health and Environment, *Health Maintenance Organizations,* Hearings on HR 5615, HR 11728 and all identical bills. Washington, DC, US Government Printing Office, 1972.

US, Congress, House, Committee on Ways and Means, *Analysis of Health Insurance Proposals Introduced in the 92nd Congress,* Committee Print. Washington, DC, US Government Printing Office, 1971.

US, Department of Health, Education, and Welfare, *Task Force on Prescription Drugs, Final Report.* Washington, DC, US Government Printing Office, 1969.

US, Department of Health, Education and Welfare: *Towards a Comprehensive Health Policy for the 1970's, A White Paper.* Washington, DC, US Government Printing Office, May 1971.

See also Congressional Hearings cited above.

## Health Services in Great Britain and Other Countries

Canada, Royal Commission on Health Services, Reports by Robert Kohn on *The Health of the Canadian People and Emerging Patterns in Health Care.* Ottawa, The Queen's Printer, 1965.

Eckstein H: *The English Health Service.* Cambridge, Massachusetts, Harvard University Press, 1958.

Evang K, Murray DS, Lear W: *Medical Care and Family Security: Norway, England, United States of America.* Englewood Cliffs, NJ, Prentice Hall, 1963.

*National Health Service Reorganization: England.* London, Her Majesty's Stationery Office, Cmd. 5055, 1972.

Farndale J, editor: *Trends in the National Health Service.* New York, MacMillan, 1964.

Forsyth, G: *Doctors and State Medicine* Philadelphia, J.B. Lippincott, 1966.

Fry, J: *Medicine in Three Societies: A Comparison of Medical Care in the USSR, USA and the UK* New York, American Elsevier, 1970.

Glaser A: *Paying the Doctor—Systems of Remuneration and Their Effects.* Baltimore, Johns Hopkins Press, 1970.

*Health Services in Britain.* New York and London, Great Britain Central Office of Information, latest edition.

*Health Services in Europe.* Copenhagen Regional Office for Europe, World Health Organization, 1965.

Hogarth J: *The Payment of the General Practitioner: Some European Comparisons.* New York, Pergamon Press, 1963.

International Labour Office: Series of Monographs on *The Organisation of Medical Care Within the Framework of Social Security*, various countries, various authors. Geneva, International Labour Office, 1968.

International Social Security Association: *Relations Between Social Security Institutions and the Medical Profession*, XIth General Meeting, Report IV. Geneva, International Social Security Association, 1953.

Lindsey A: *Socialized Medicine in England and Wales: The National Health Service, 1948-1961*. Chapel Hill, University of North Carolina Press, 1962.

Mencher S: *British Private Medical Practice and the National Health Service*. Pittsburgh, University of Pittsburgh Press, 1968.

Roemer MI: *The Organisation of Medical Care Under Social Security*. Geneva, International Labour Office, 1969.

Stevens R: *Medical Practice in Modern England: The Impact of Specialisation and State Medicine*. New Haven, Yale University Press, 1966.

*The British National Health Service*. Chicago, American College of Hospital Administrators, 1969.

# Periodicals

The following periodicals devote considerable attention to developments, problems and policy issues in the health services. Where the sponsoring organization is not self-evident from the title, this is indicated in brackets.

*American Journal of Public Health* (American Public Health Association).

*American Journal of Nursing* (reflecting views of the American Nurses Association).

*Bulletin of the New York Academy of Medicine.*

*Group Health and Welfare News* (Journal of the Group Health Association of America).

*HEALTH/PAC Bulletin* (publication of the Health Policy Advisory Center).

*HSMHA Health Reports* (a continuation of *Public Health Reports*, official journal of the Health Services and Mental Health Administration, US Department of Health, Education, and Welfare).

*Hospital Administration* (a publication of the American College of Hospital Administrators).

*Hospitals: Journal of the American Hospital Association.*

*Inquiry: A Journal of Medical Care Organization, Provision and Financing* (a publication of the Blue Cross Association).

*International Social Security Review* (formerly *Bulletin of the International Social Security Association*).

*JAMA* (Journal of the American Medical Association).

*Journal of Health and Social Behavior* (a publication of the American Sociological Association).

*Lancet* (London, England; independent).

*Medical Care* (an international journal sponsored by the Medical Care Section of the American Public Health Association).

*Medical Care Review* (a publication of the Bureau of Public Health Economics School of Public Health, University of Michigan).

*New England Journal of Medicine* (published by the Massachusetts Medical Society).

*Nursing Outlook* (reflecting views of the National League for Nursing).

*The Milbank Memorial Fund Quarterly.*

*The Physicians' Forum.*

*Social Security Bulletin* (official publication of the Office of Research and Statistics of the Social Security Administration, US Department of Health, Education, and Welfare).

*Welare in Reivew* (official publication of the Social and Rehabilitation Service, US Department of Health, Education and Welfare).

The periodic publications of the US National Center for Health Statistics, US Department of Health, Education, and Welfare, should be consulted for statistical data.